A Mammographers Guide: Radiological and Histopathological Guidelines

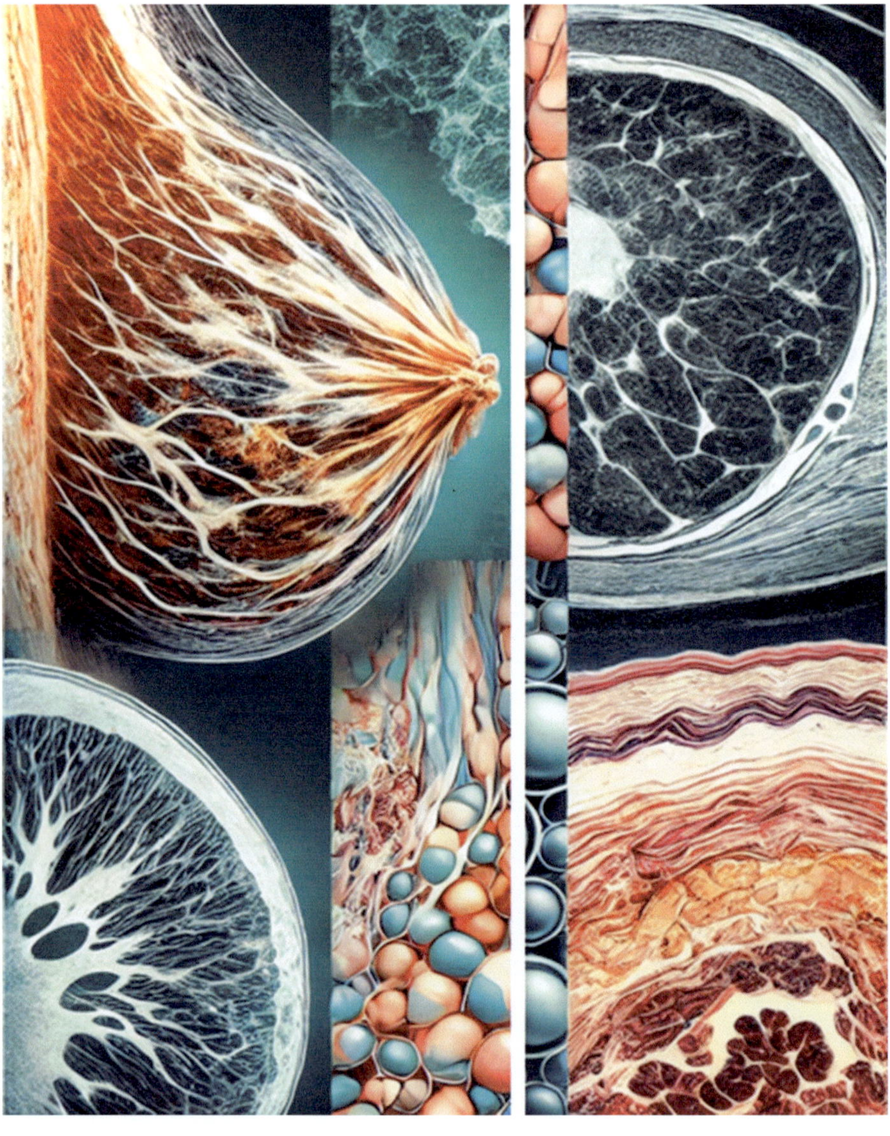

Kathryn Malherbe

A Mammographers Guide: Radiological and Histopathological Guidelines

Springer

Kathryn Malherbe
Malherbe Imaging Inc
Pretoria, Gauteng, South Africa

ISBN 978-3-031-84666-3 ISBN 978-3-031-84667-0 (eBook)
https://doi.org/10.1007/978-3-031-84667-0

This Springer imprint is published by the registered company Springer Nature Switzerland AG
The registered company address is: Gewerbestrasse 11, 6330 Cham, Switzerland

Contents

List of Figures

List of Tables

Imaging of Breast Pathology

1

Contents

K. Malherbe, *A Mammographers Guide: Radiological and Histopathological Guidelines*, https://doi.org/10.1007/978-3-031-84667-0_1

In the field of breast imaging, when patients present with clinically palpable lumps or other visual indicators suggestive of malignancy, it is essential to follow a standard imaging protocol to ensure optimal imaging quality. The initial imaging typically includes cranial-caudal (CC) and mediolateral oblique (MLO) views, which are the primary modalities for detecting potential pathological findings. Subsequently, the mammographer assesses the bilateral or unilateral breast tissue and compares the current imaging with previous studies to identify any new densities [1–4].

If a density is noted in the far upper outer quadrant, an exaggerated lateral CC view can be performed (see Fig. 1.1). When the density is not concordant between the CC and MLO views, a mediolateral (ML) view can be used to assist in localizing the density in a 90-degree plane.

For masses located near the chest wall or sternum, a cleavage view or exaggerated medial CC view may be employed. Other specialized views, such as rolled CC or MLO views, are useful when a density is observed only in one of these standard views. For example, if a density is noted only on the lateral aspect of the CC view, the tissue can be rolled medially (upper surface) and laterally (lower skin surface) to determine if the density is indeed solid or merely superimposed tissue (see Figs. 1.2 and 1.3) [5].

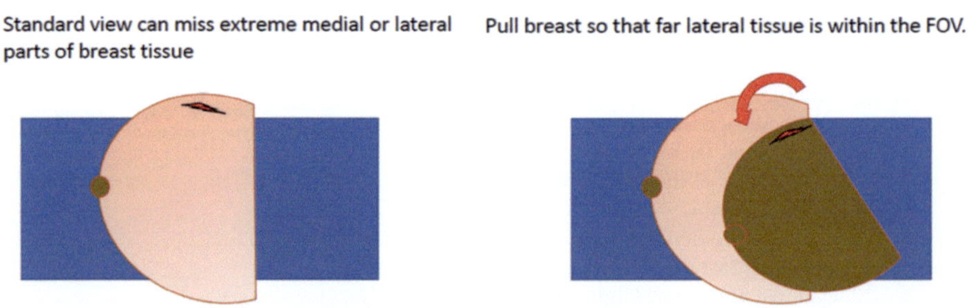

Fig. 1.1 Standard vs. exaggerated lateral view

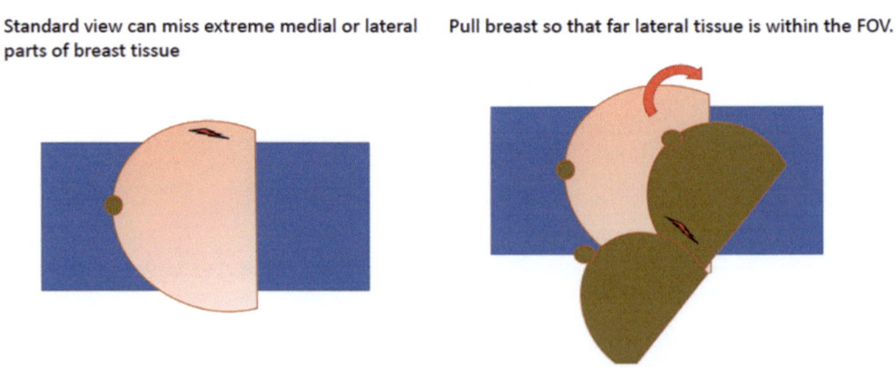

Fig. 1.2 Standard vs. exaggerated medial view

Fig. 1.3 Example of a hidden group of calcifications seen with exaggerated medial CC view

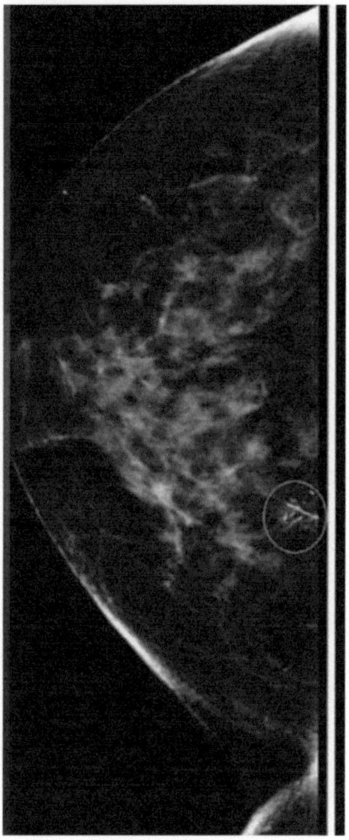

Similarly, for the MLO view, if a density is observed only in the upper part of the breast, and not as well on the CC view (as noted in Fig. 1.4), the tissue can be rolled superiorly (anterior skin surface) and inferiorly (posterior skin surface closest to the image receptor) to ascertain if the density is genuine or superimposed fibroglandular tissue [6].

In Fig. 1.5, a region of dense overlapped tissue is only seen on the CC view, the mammographer then places their own hand on the top skin surface, and the other under the breast surface. The top hand then rolls the superior tissue laterally and the bottom hand rolls in the opposite direction. If it is only superimposed tissue, the resultant image should show the area as less dense. If, however, it remains as is, ultrasound imaging is prompted to further investigate.

For patients with breast prostheses, Eklund views are crucial to reveal any hidden lesions in the retromammary space, which are often missed during standard CC and MLO imaging.

Other important considerations include the use of optimal exposure techniques, such as increasing the kilovoltage peak (KVP) by 2 or the milliampere-seconds (mAs) by 15% if a mass is very dense and standard exposure values are insufficient for adequate penetration. Magnification views are also employed to enlarge regions with fine microcalcifications or to spread out dense areas of tissue if the previously mentioned rolled views are inconclusive.

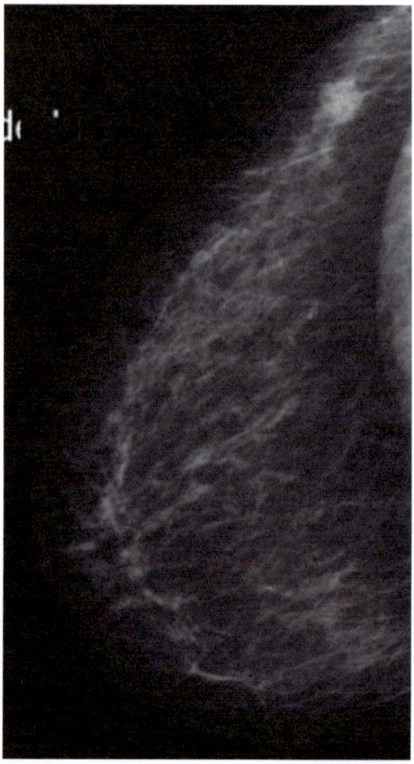

Fig. 1.4 An example of a hidden density seen with exaggerated lateral CC view

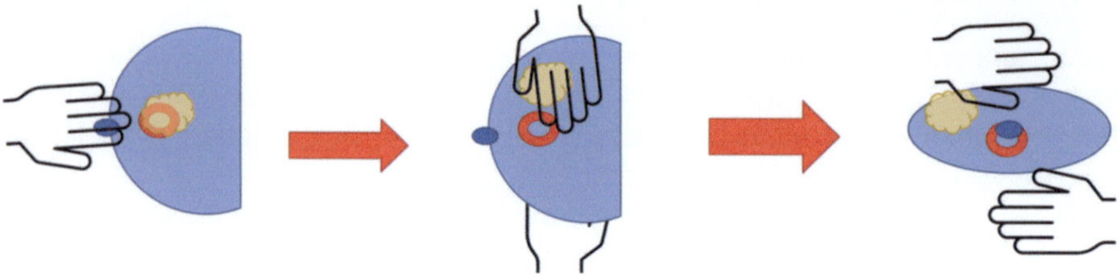

Fig. 1.5 Example of rolled view

A lesser common special view to use for kyphotic or male patients to be able to perform the CC view is the From Below view (FB view). For this the entire mammogram C-arm is rotated with the purpose of scooping up breast tissue from below and then avoiding shadowing from an encroached shoulder or patient having very little breast tissue present, making pulling over of tissue difficult [1, 7, 8].

Fig. 1.6 demonstrates the concept of a from below view; however from a practical point of view, it requires the mammographer to be crouched down on their knees to be able to view the inferior breast tissue and to ensure all is seen on the resultant image

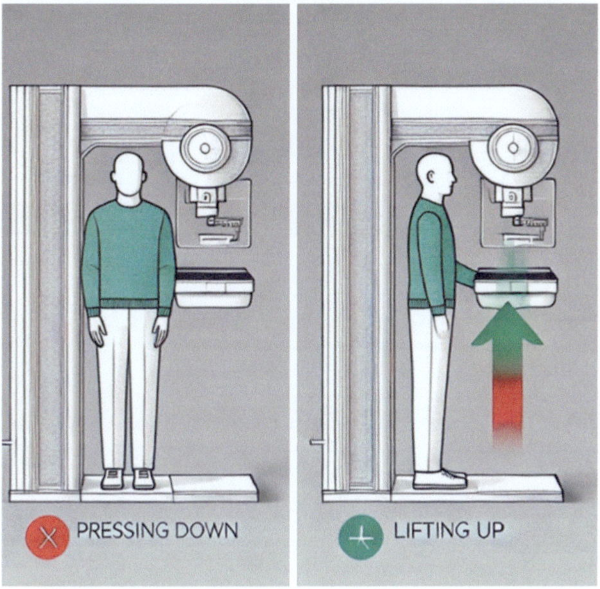

Fig. 1.6 Example from below view for a male patient
The image receptor is turned 180 degrees so that a scooping action is promoted by means of the compression paddle, from below to ensure a maximum amount of breast tissue is gathered for the view

Beyond the imaging process, a mammographer must prioritize patient care and communication throughout investigative imaging. It is essential to inform patients before the standard mammogram that additional views may be necessary to further evaluate dense tissue regions and that this should not be a cause for concern. By preparing patients in this way, they are less likely to be anxious if additional imaging is required.

When uncertainty arises regarding an area of interest, additional imaging should be considered. The instinct of a mammographer often leads to the detection of occult disease that might be overlooked by standard diagnostic procedures [9, 10]

1.1 Physics in Mammography

The goal of mammography is to provide sufficient contrast differences between normal soft tissue structures and a breast lesion (Fig. 1.7). Different structures in the breast have variance in attenuation properties. The depicted contrast on an image is produced by x-rays transmitting through various soft tissue structures of varying densities. X-ray attenuation coefficients of normal soft tissue and malignancy are similar in mammographic appearance. For this reason, to avoid detection errors, low-energy x-rays are used.

1.1.1 Conventional Screen Film Mammography

There are many limitations to the use of screen films in mammography due to the advances in latest imaging techniques surpassing the imaging capabilities of screen film mammography (see Table 1.1).

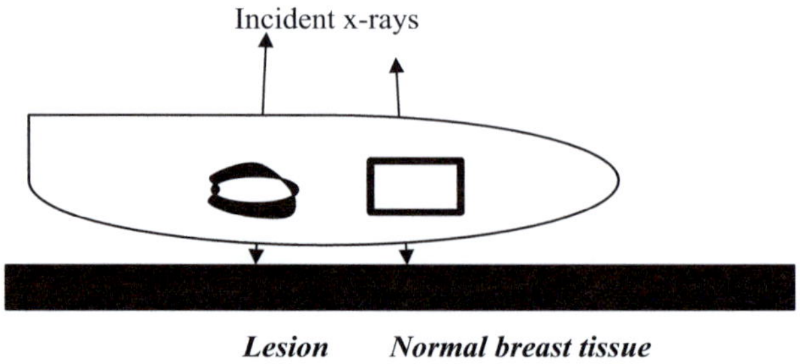

Fig. 1.7 Incident x-ray beam during mammographic imaging

Table 1.1 Various characteristics related to digital systems (see Fig. 1.10)

Phosphor flat panel detector	Phosphor CCD
Amorphous silicon (see Fig. 1.13) plate with a rectangular array of light-sensitive photodiodes X-rays are absorbed by the thallium layer which activates cesium iodide phosphor onto photodiodes (dels) The dels detect light emitted by phosphor to produce an electric signal stored on each del	CSiTi phosphor deposited onto a coupling plate with optical fibers Serves 2 functions: Conduct light from phosphor plate Protects CCD from diagnostic exposure to x-rays. Disadvantages: Longer image acquisition time X-ray tube heat load is higher Advantages: No grid required due to less scatter absorption Less expensive
Computed radiography	**Selenium flat panel detectors**
Photostimulable phosphor screens, more commonly known as CR, have been used for many years in general radiography as well in digital mammography. The basic principle of CR systems is "photostimulable luminescence." energy from x-rays is absorbed in a screen composed of phosphor material containing a high prevalence of electron trapping sites. The absorbed energy frees electrons in the phosphor crystal for a short period to time within the crystal lattice where they are stored. The analog image is then read by placing the screen in a reading device and scanned by a red laser beam. This causes the electrons to be freed and to return to their original state within the crystal lattice. The gain affects both the sensitivity and noise of imaging systems. Inadequate amounts of light will cause additional noise above the typical quantum noise, causing the SNR and DQE to reduce. Manufacturers have overcome this by allowing the laser reader to read both the top and bottom surfaces of the phosphor plate to increase the efficiency of light collection and to reduce laser scattering	X-rays are absorbed by a thin layer of amorphous selenium. X-rays interact with selenium to produce energetic photoelectrons, which lose their kinetic energy during interactions with electrons in the outer orbitals of selenium atoms. The process of electrons being freed produces holes during the departure, known as "electron-hole pairs" which form the signal. An electric field is applied between electrodes deposited on the upper and lower surfaces of the selenium as it sweeps an electric charge toward the electrodes. The dels act as capacitors to store the charge. At the corner of each del is a TFT switch. The readout of each del occurs in a similar fashion as with phosphor flat panel detectors with control lines activating the TFTs in a sequential manner [14, 15]

The disadvantages of screen film mammography are:

- Nonlinearity and saturation response of the films.
  - Saturation refers to the lack of optical density changes postprocessing.
  - All silver halide molecules are used during initial image formation.
- Inability of postprocessing.
  - That is, brightness and contrast.
- Quantum noise due to incomplete absorption of x-rays by screen.
- Granular content of film emulsion.
- Increased rate of scatter radiation.

Comparative performance techniques used for digital mammography include:

- Modular transfer function is measured as spatial resolution. It assesses limiting resolution as line pairs/mm from a set bar pattern.
- Detective quantum efficiency.
- SNR quality of image; as the SNR increases, exposure values increase [11].

1.1.2 Digital Mammography

Allows optimization in image acquisition, storage, processing, and display capabilities (see Fig. 1.8).

1.1.3 Properties of Digital Images

- Spatial resolution is affected by the size of del, effective focal spot size, magnification, spread of signal, motion, and type of breast tissue/detector.
- Detector element size refers to a set of detectors elements.

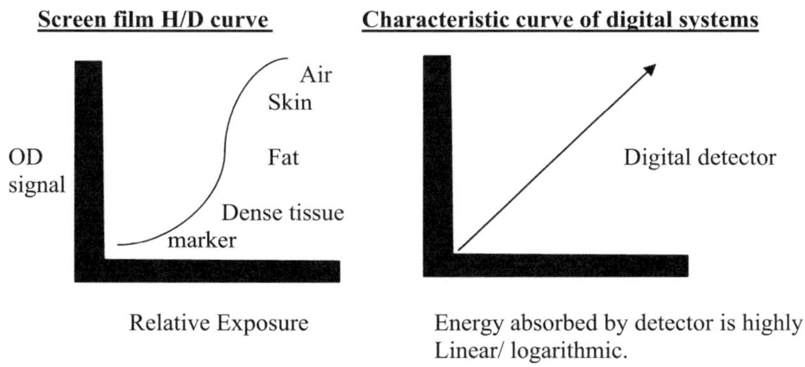

Fig. 1.8 Characteristic curve of screen film vs. digital mammography systems

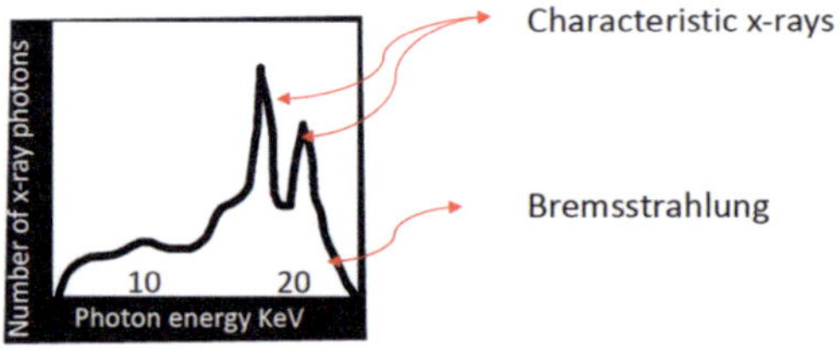

Fig. 1.9 Energy spectra

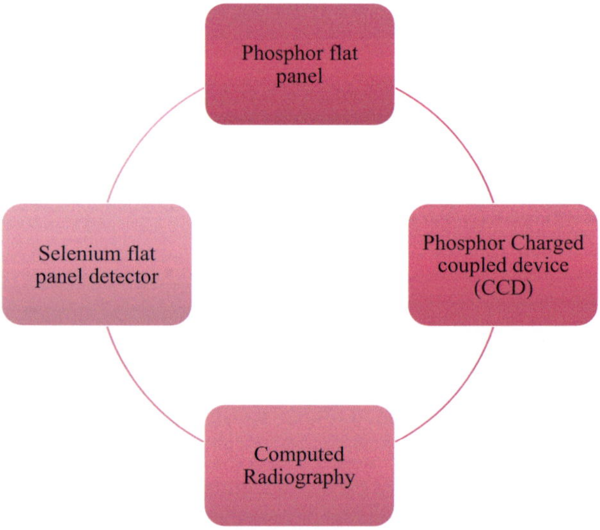

Fig. 1.10 Various types of detectors in digital imaging

- Dynamic range refers to the range of intensities recorded. Determine by the number of bits and the x-ray fluence. Range should have adequate response for unattenuated x-ray beam at the edge of the breast tissue surface.
- Energy spectra refer to the number of photons (see Fig. 1.9) [12, 13].

1.1.4 Types of Digital Systems

Characteristic x-rays refer to certain x-ray photons being generated within a specific energy range of characteristics. Interactions between accelerated electrons and the atoms of the anode produce "characteristic x-rays" as they are generated according to the material which they generate from. For a characteristic x-ray to be generated, accelerated electrons must have sufficient energy to knock out an electron in one of the outer shells of the atom. The loss of an electron produces an unstable situation. The displaced electron is replaced by another of the atom's electrons from a higher energy level. As the electron moves from its higher energy level to a lower energy level, a surge of energy is released in the form of an x-ray photon (see Fig. 1.11). Since the atom produced relates to the atomic nr of the atom and the energy levels

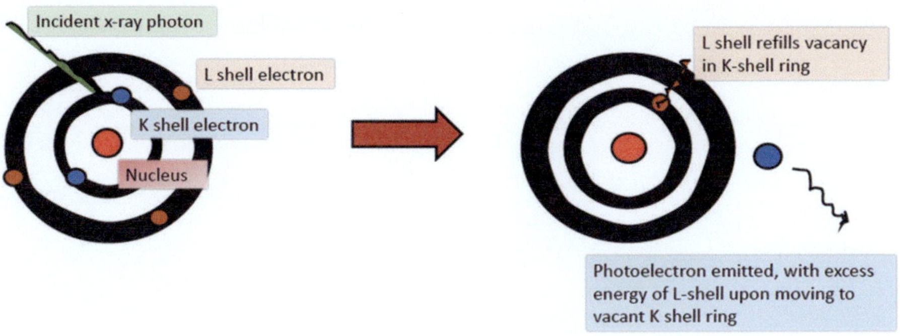

Fig. 1.11 Schematic representation of the photoelectric effect

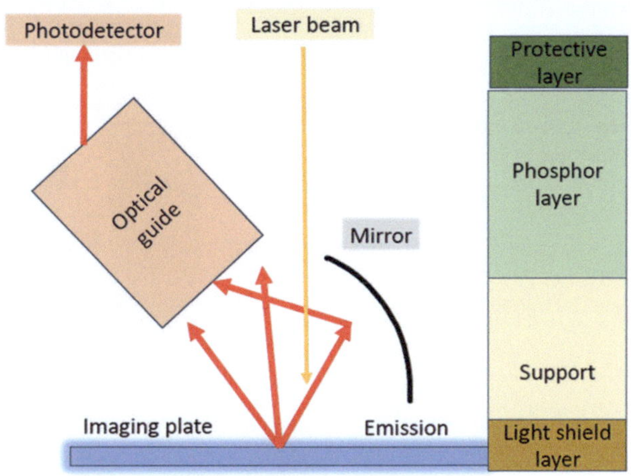

Fig. 1.12 Photostimulable phosphor system

between the electrons moving, the x-ray photons are "characteristic" of the atom which generated it [15, 16].

Spatial resolution decreases as the detector thickness increases. In an ideal setting, all emitted light would arise from the point of x-ray interaction (see Fig. 1.12), but scattering of the readout laser light within the phosphor material causes blur.

The quality of x-rays produced, and characteristic energy output depend on the anode material used such as molybdenum, rhodium, and tungsten. Molybdenum is typically in the 17 KeV range, Rhodium in the 20.2 KeV range, and Tungsten has an emission range of 59 KeV. Digital detectors work more efficiently with a Tungsten anode material since it has a higher tolerance for heated focal spots. More heat tolerant tubes allow higher energy photons, faster exposure times, and improved imaging with digital detectors.

The key principle of mammographic imaging is the production of high-resolution images to depict fine morphological structures such as microcalcifications. To reach this purpose, the focal spot in a mammographic system is a key component. The focal spot is the area on the anode where the electrons (accelerated from the

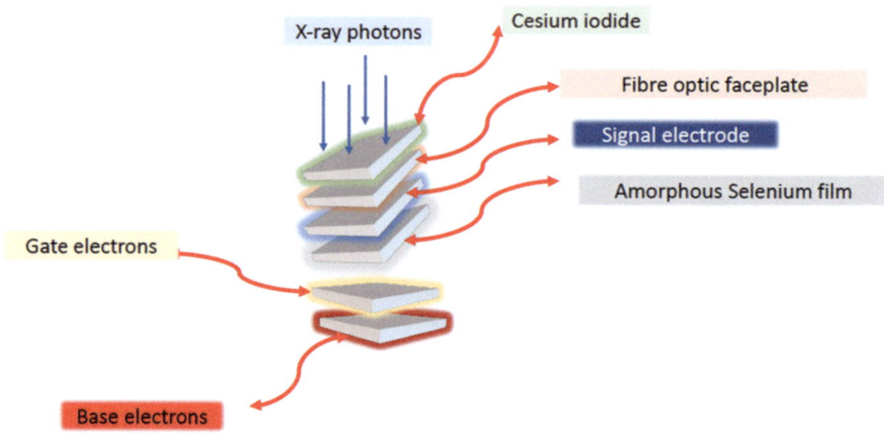

Fig. 1.13 Amorphous selenium flat panel detector schematic drawing

Fig. 1.14 Line focus principle

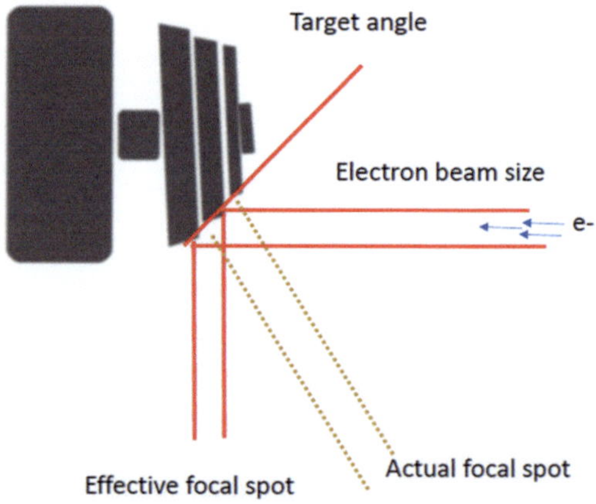

cathode) strike the anode. This also caused the production of heat. The design of focal spots is such to have it as small as possible in size but can also produce many photons over a short period of time. For this reason, the actual focal spot is larger than the effective focal spot. This means that the geometric sharpness of the image varies also over various parts of the breast.

The Line Focus Principle (see Figs. 1.13 and 1.14) is a description of electron interaction with the anode and direction change. The three main purposes are:

- To direct x-ray photons toward the patient/ breast tissue.
- To angle the target material for a smaller effective focal spot size.
- To narrow the beam for increased resolution [8, 17, 18]

In screen/film imaging, adequate breast compression is required for a narrow exposure latitude and high contrast resolution in the produced image. Due to the cone-shaped nature of the breast, compression is required to produce an evenly compressed region of interest. This allows a uniform exposure to be obtained. Since the dynamic range of digital systems is so broad, exposure latitude and variations in exposure values can be automatically corrected in digital systems. This allows for less compression of breast tissue but can be affected by other factors such as scatter and spread of overlapping fibroglandular breast tissue [19].

Why Do We Use Breast Compression?

- To hold the breast away from the chest wall, allowing projection of breast tissue without interference of noise from adjacent thorax structures.
- To reduce blur due to motion by physically holding the breast immobilized.
- To reduce the dose due to decreased breast thickness and attenuation.
- To reduce dose and motion due to shorter exposure time.
- To separate overlapping structures for improved accuracy.
- To reduce blur and geometric sharpness by bringing relevant structures closer to the detector surface.
- To reduce image scatter.
- To produce uniform thickness and exposure outputs.
- Allows accurate registration of images for computer reconstruction algorithms.

The x-ray image is formed by differential absorption of photons passing through the breast and various soft tissue structures. Certain overlapping shadows are cast on the detector, depending on the path which the photons travelled to reach the detector. Most x-ray interactions at the energy levels of mammographic imaging involve photoelectric absorption in which an x-ray photon is completely absorbed by displacing an electron. This produces image sharpness [20, 21].

Another form of x-ray interaction is Compton scattering (see Fig. 1.15). The photon transfers a portion of its energy to an electron. The photon continues its path out of the atom, but the direction of its path is changed. Many of these interactions move in incoherent pathways, which leads to increased image sharpness. The secondary photons produced by scatter radiation significantly affects the image quality in mammography [11].

Due to x-ray divergence, magnification is obtained by placing the object closer to the focal spot and further away from the detector surface. Magnification methods use small focal spots, since large focal spots will increase geometric blur and decrease overall spatial resolution. Magnification helps to "spread out" structures over an increased number of imaging "dels," which allows improved differentiation of structures. In digital systems, overall SNR, dose, and exposure time are increased by using magnification.

Due to the breast being placed closer to the focal spot, the photons exiting the breast are spread over a larger area, thus requiring increased dose. The electron beam deriving from the cathode is concentrated over a smaller portion of the focal

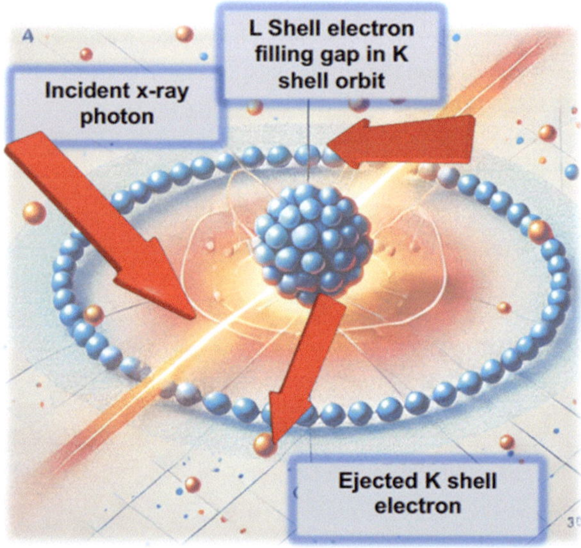

Fig. 1.15 Compton Scattering diagram

spot causing increased heat being generated. For this reason the mA output must be reduced from 90–150 mAs to 30–40 mAs [19].

1.2 Image Interpretation in Mammography

Detection refers to the process of finding anomalies of which most are proven malignant. Diagnosis is the ability to characterize an anomaly as benign or malignant [7].

Screening is a systematic evaluation process for detection of unsuspected disease.

Diagnostic mammography is most effective when used as part of a screening evaluation in asymptomatic women. Over 60% of palpable masses are not evident on mammography, the major role of mammography is to detect the clinically nonpalpable anomalies of the breast.

Prevalence is the number of cancers in a population at a given time, whereas incidence is the number of cancers diagnosed each year after a prevalence screen. Positive predictive value (PPV) is the measure of the discriminating power of the method being analyzed. This is determined as the number of true cancers divided by the number of tests called positive for cancer. PPV can also be used for biopsy accuracy by determining the number of cancers diagnosed by the number of lesions recommended for biopsy. Sensitivity is a measure of a diagnostic test's ability to find cancers in a population. It is calculated as the nr of cancers correctly diagnosed by the test divided by the nr of cancers present in the population. Specificity is a measure of how successful a screening test is at saying cancer is present when it really is not present. A good screening program will detect 40–50% of cancers under the size of 1 cm or smaller in diameter per annum. Six to ten cancers per 1000 women screened should be detected [18, 22].

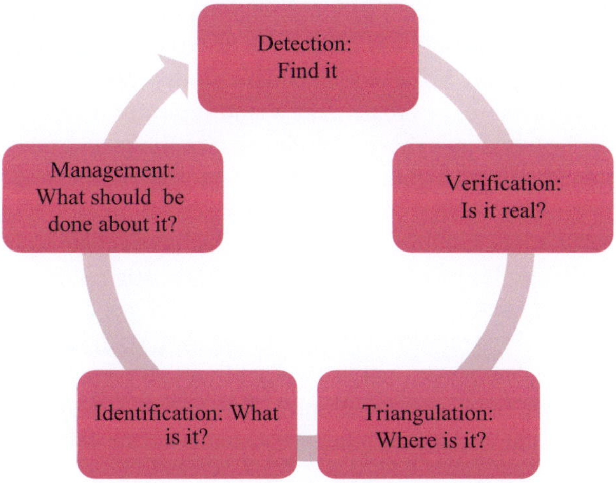

Fig. 1.16 Systematic imaging approach

A systematic approach:

If a mass has uncertain positioning, factors such as skin markers or localization grid can be used to identify its position (see Fig. 1.16). Rolled views also aid in determining whether the lesion is in the upper or lower half of the compressed breast as well as to confirm the depicted lesion is a solid mass or overlapping breast tissue simulating a breast mass.

A straight lateral projection can be used to assess a mass which is only on the oblique view. The shift of the lesion relative to the projection of breast tissues can be used to determine its location in the breast [23].

1.2.1 Screening and Diagnostic Mammography

Mammography remains the cornerstone of breast cancer screening, with its utility spanning both screening and diagnostic purposes. Screening mammography is used as a preventative measure in asymptomatic women, aiming to detect early-stage cancers, while diagnostic mammography is employed when a patient presents with symptoms such as palpable lumps, pain, or abnormal findings on other imaging modalities [4, 7, 17, 22, 32–37]. The role of mammographers is crucial in both contexts, as they ensure the accurate acquisition of high-quality images, assist in patient positioning, and work closely with radiologists to optimize diagnostic accuracy.

In screening mammography, patients are typically asymptomatic women who meet the age and risk criteria for regular screenings. For instance, women aged 50–74 with no prior history of breast cancer and no current symptoms are commonly referred for biennial screenings, as recommended by the U.S. Preventive Services Task Force [1]. Additionally, women at higher risk, such as those with a family history of breast cancer, may begin screening earlier, starting as young as 40, or even younger for those with genetic predispositions like BRCA1 or BRCA2 mutations [2].

In contrast, diagnostic mammography is reserved for women who present with specific breast-related symptoms or who have abnormal findings from a screening mammogram. For example, a patient who reports discovering a palpable lump, nipple discharge, or breast pain would typically be referred for diagnostic imaging to further evaluate these symptoms. Similarly, if a screening mammogram reveals abnormalities such as asymmetric density or microcalcifications, diagnostic mammography is used to obtain more detailed images and aid in determining whether further investigation, such as a biopsy, is necessary.

Examples of patients requiring diagnostic mammography include a 45-year-old woman with a newly discovered lump in her breast or a 55-year-old who notices spontaneous nipple discharge. In contrast, a 52-year-old asymptomatic woman with no significant personal or family history of breast cancer would likely undergo routine screening mammography. This differentiation ensures appropriate care pathways and allows for the early detection of breast cancer, which is critical for improving patient outcomes [3, 4, 36, 37].

The discrepancies in screening guidelines and access across countries further influence the frequency and utilization of screening versus diagnostic mammography. In the United States, where routine screening is widely implemented, asymptomatic women are often regularly referred for screenings. Meanwhile, in countries with limited resources, like South Africa, diagnostic mammography might play a larger role, as women often present with more advanced symptoms due to delayed screenings.

However, the approaches to mammography screening vary significantly across countries. For example, in the United States, mammographic screening is widely recommended for women aged 40 and above, with biennial screening starting at age 50, as suggested by the U.S. Preventive Services Task Force (USPSTF) [7]. In contrast, the United Kingdom's NHS Breast Screening Programme invites women aged 50–70 for mammography every 3 years [37]. Meanwhile, in countries like South Africa, mammographic screening is not yet a nationwide initiative, and access is often limited to urban areas, with rural women being under-screened due to resource constraints [38]. The discrepancies in screening guidelines and access highlight the diverse challenges mammographers face in different settings, further underscoring the need for context-specific strategies in breast cancer detection.

1.2.2 Distribution of Calcifications

The distribution of calcifications, as seen in Table 1.2, are arranged according to the risk of malignancy (See Figs. 1.17, 1.18, 1.19, and 1.20):

- Diffuse: distributed randomly throughout the breast.
- Regional: occupying a large portion of breast tissue >2 cm greatest dimension.
- Grouped (historically cluster): few calcifications occupying a small portion of breast tissue: lower limit 5 calcifications within 1 cm and upper limit a larger number of calcifications within 2 cm.

Table 1.2 BIRADS feature analysis [2, 5, 39, 40]

Suspicious morphology	
So small and/or hazy in appearance that a more specific particle shape cannot be determined.	**Amorphous** (BI-RADS 4B)
Irregular, conspicuous calcifications that are generally between 0.5 mm and 1 mm and tend to coalesce but are smaller than dystrophic calcifications	**Coarse and heterogeneous** (BI-RADS 4B)
Usually, more conspicuous than amorphous forms and are seen to have discrete shapes, without fine-linear and linear branching forms, usually <0.5 mm	**Fine pleomorphic** (BI-RADS 4C)
Thin, linear irregular calcifications, may be discontinuous, occasionally branching forms can be seen, usually <0.5 mm	**Fine linear or fine-linear branching** (BI-RADS 4C)
Typically benign	
Skin, vascular, coarse, large rod like, round or punctate (< 1 mm), rim, dystrophic, milk of calcium and suture calcifications are typically benign	
There is one exception of the rule: An isolated group of punctuate calcifications that is new, increasing, linear, or segmental in distribution, or adjacent to a known cancer can be assigned as probably benign or suspicious	

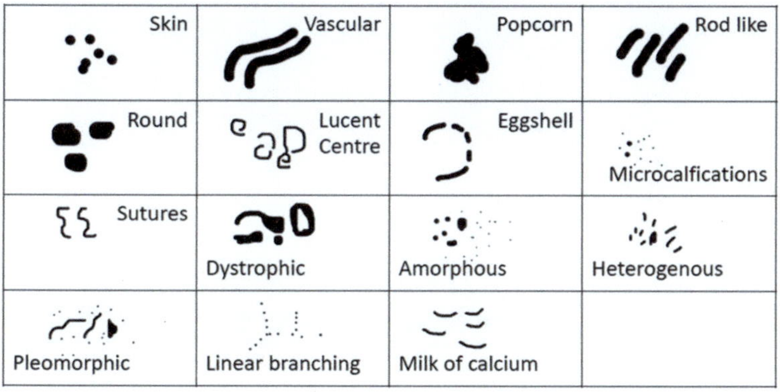

Fig. 1.17 Classification of calcifications in mammography

- Linear: arranged in a line, which suggests deposits in a duct.
- Segmental: suggests deposits in a duct or ducts and their branches [31]

1.2.3 Calcifications

A mass seen on a mammogram image can frequently be deduced by any associated calcifications. A mass with large, popcorn-like calcifications is typically associated with a benign involuting fibroadenoma or less commonly a papilloma. Fine, curvilinear calcifications which surround an oval mass are most likely related to a benign cyst. Pleomorphic calcifications smaller than 0.5 mm and associated with or without a mass are inferred as suspicious findings. These types of calcifications occur in the intraductal component of a mixed lesion. The presence of calcifications within

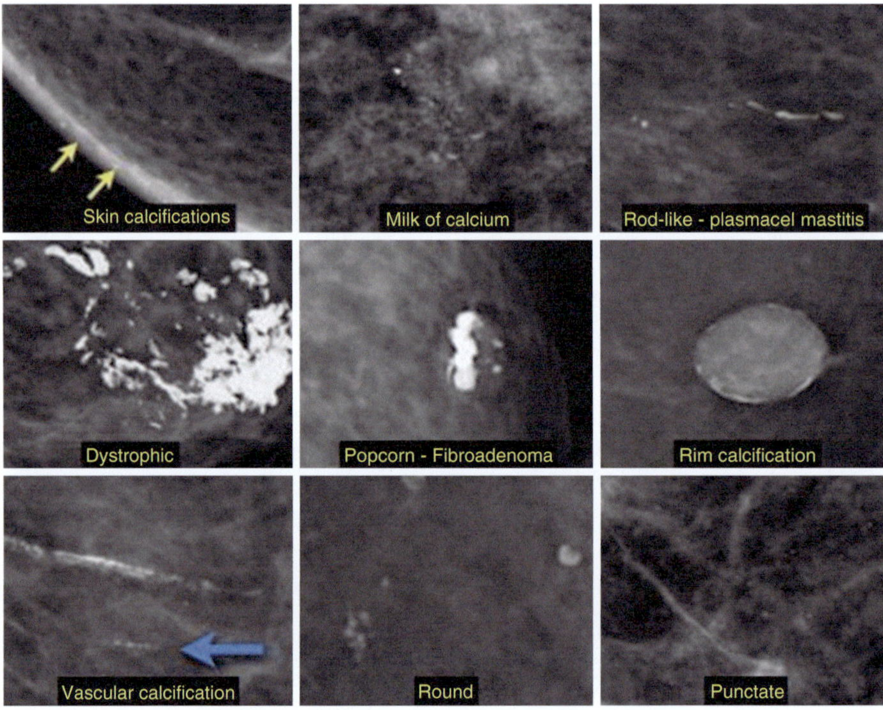

Fig. 1.18 Benign calcifications on mammography [24]

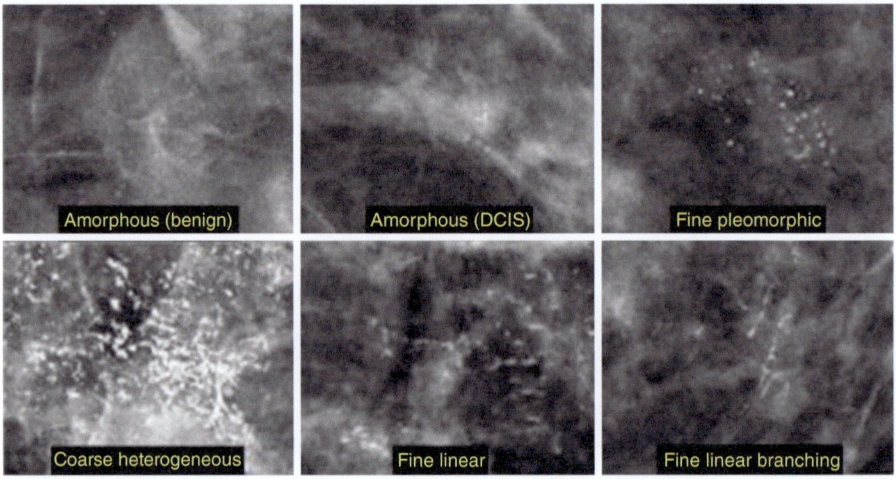

Fig. 1.19 Suspicious type findings of calcifications [25–30]

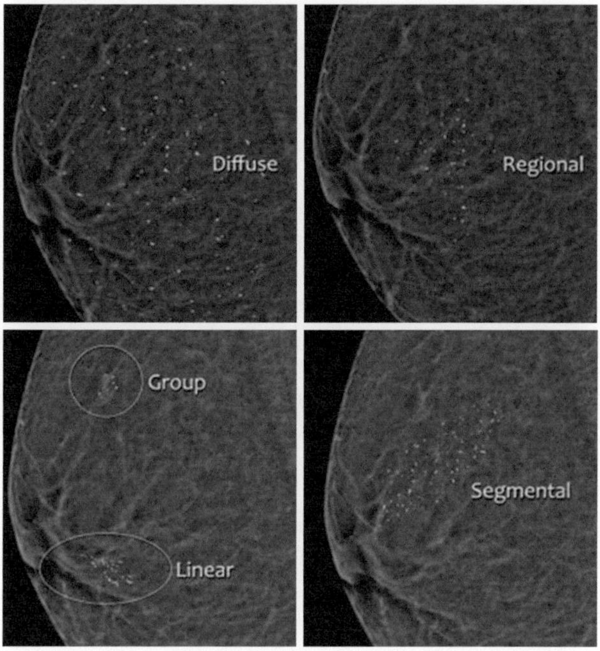

Fig. 1.20 Types of distributions of calcifications [31]

lesions already appearing malignant in morphological appearance increases the likelihood of cancer.

Calcium deposits are frequently found in the breast. Some forms of calcium deposits occur due to active cell secretion or due to necrotic cellular debris. This may be in response to inflammation, trauma, radiation, or foreign bodies. Calcifications can be located in or outside ducts, lobular acini, vascular structures, interlobar stroma, fat, and in the skin.

When assessing calcifications, the size, location, number, and distribution are important factors [5].

1.2.4 Other Associated Findings

Skin, nipple, trabecular changes, and axillary adenopathy are all features involved in the assessment of mammographic abnormality.

The skin forms the outer envelope of the breast, and the epidermal layer is in direct contact with the ductal epithelium as it descends from the nipple to the duct orifices. This is believed to be the route of spread of ductal carcinoma onto the nipple as Paget's disease. The average breast thickness is around 3 mm and changes in the value can relate to abnormal findings.

Thickening of the skin can have many causes and can be focal, diffuse, unilateral, or bilateral. The causes thereof vary from tumor invasion, tumor in dermal lymphatics, lymphatic congestion, or even congestive heart failure. Major differential diagnoses for skin changes include malignancy, infection, inflammation, psoriasis, lymphatic obstruction as well as systemic diseases such as scleroderma [2, 41, 42].

Nipple discharges are a common occurrence. Discharges can vary from milky, yellow, green, brown, clear, and bloody. Bilateral breast discharges are typically due to central hormonal causes. Most unilateral breast discharges are related to benign disease. If the discharge is unilateral and from a solitary duct, a mass is suspected, such as a large duct papilloma which are benign hyperplastic growths with a fibrovascular core [6, 26, 43].

Axillary lymph nodes allow lymphatic drainage of the breast to channels such as the internal mammary chain. Spread of a tumor to the axillary lymph nodes is indicative of the tumors biological probability of metastasis and prognostic rates. Normal axillary lymph nodes are less than 2 cm in size and present with a typical hilar notch or lucent center [44].

1.2.5 The Altered Breast Appearance

Various factors can affect the clinical and radiological appearance of breast tissue such as pregnancy, lactation, abscess, biopsy, mastectomy, radiation, and implants.

During pregnancy, the initial imaging for any palpable mass should be ultrasound, to reduce radiation exposure risk to the unborn fetus. Since lactation has not yet occurred, the breast tissue is not overtly dense during imaging, and if necessary, on case-by-case basis and proper informed consent has been obtained, mammography can be performed during pregnancy.

During lactation there is vast amplification and multiplication of breast lobules with an increase in fat droplets within the epithelial cytoplasm. The intralobular stroma reduces and is replaced by multiple enlarged lobules. During onset of lactation, significant secretions from the acini are produced. This causes an increased density of the breast tissue, limiting mammographic sensitivity [45].

A breast abscess is a common occurrence in the breast clinic, with patients presenting with erythema, swelling and tenderness as the initial clinical symptomatology. The typical sonographic findings are skin thickening, increased echogenicity of the fibroglandular breast tissue along with increased hyperemia when Color Doppler or Power Doppler imaging is used [6, 46].

Following core needle biopsy, the breast tissue undergoes hematoma formation, resorption, and fibrous tissue developing as part of the healing process. This can cause certain discrepancies during follow-up examinations, as malignant masses tend to have a similar dense fibrotic appearance on ultrasound. For this reason, short-term follow-up is always suggested, or skin markers/biopsy markers should be utilized in situ, to confirm a stable mammographic and sonographic appearance. Coarse calcifications can also develop long term following surgical biopsy intervention, and these are typically part of the healing process causing fat necrosis. Annual follow-up examination would include assessment with previous findings to ensure no associated pleomorphic fine calcifications develop adjacent to the previous region of interest [32, 44, 47–49].

Mastectomy or breast reduction surgery (mammaplasty) also causes significant changes in the imaging appearance of breast tissue. It is important to understand the method of intervention and the changes which typically occur to be able to distinguish benign and malignant findings. Radiation therapy typically causes skin thickening and changes of the internal architecture of any excess breast parenchyma. Six-month follow-up imaging studies are typically suggested during the treatment period [38, 50, 51].

1.2.6 Appearance of the Male Breast

From 1% to 2% of all breast cancers are male patients. The referral of a male patient for a mammogram or ultrasound is due to the patient or his referring physician feeling an asymmetric thickening, focal nipple tenderness, and swelling or there is overall breast enlargement. The most common finding or result is gynecomastia. Often, the contralateral, asymptomatic breast would also present with gynecomastia, but to a lesser extent.

At birth, male breast tissue has a similar anatomical appearance with subareolar ducts like prepubertal girls. When certain hormonal factors or hypertensive drugs are used by a male, the ducts can undergo differentiation and elongation, and however limited lobular growth is seen. Because these ductal components of men contain ductal epithelium, there is a slight risk of carcinoma development. Gynecomastia refers to nonneoplastic enlargement of the male breast [9, 10, 52]. Clinically the breast presents as firm, enlarged tissue in the retroareolar complex with associated edema a common finding. No studies have proven that the incidence of gynecomastia increased the lifetime risk of an individual to develop cancer. Gynecomastia's onset can be from numerous factors such as endogenous hormonal imbalances, hormone-producing tumors, hepatic disease, renal disease, and hyperthyroidism. Various blood pressure medication has also been shown with studies to be associated with the development of gynecomastia. In adolescents, transient changes are common and are usually self-limiting and regress as normal hormonal activity stabilizes. Drugs such as reserpine, cardiac glycosides, spironolactone, cimetidine, thiazides, and marijuana have been associated with gynecomastia. Klinefelter's syndrome has also been associated with an increased risk for breast cancer.

Mammographic evaluation would include bilateral MLO and adjunct ultrasound evaluation.

1.2.7 BIRADS and US-BIRADS Lexicon

The Breast Imaging Reporting and Data System (BI-RADS) is a standardized lexicon developed by the American College of Radiology (ACR) to categorize breast imaging findings and their associated risk of malignancy. It provides uniformity in reporting and facilitates clear communication between radiologists, referring physicians, and patients. The BI-RADS lexicon applies primarily to mammography, ultrasound, and MRI, helping guide management decisions based on specific descriptors and classifications of breast lesions. The US-BIRADS lexicon specifically refers to its use in breast ultrasound imaging and includes similar standardizations to ensure accurate and consistent reporting [31].

The BI-RADS lexicon comprises categories 0 through 6, each indicating a specific level of suspicion for malignancy. Category 0 indicates an incomplete evaluation, necessitating additional imaging, while Category 1 represents a negative finding with no abnormalities detected. Category 2 denotes benign findings, such as simple cysts, and requires routine follow-up. Categories 3–5 represent varying degrees of suspicion, with Category 3 suggesting a probably benign finding that requires short-term follow-up, Category 4 indicating a suspicious abnormality warranting biopsy, and Category 5 denoting a highly suspicious finding with a strong likelihood of malignancy. Finally, Category 6 is reserved for cases where a biopsy-proven malignancy has already been confirmed.

The US-BIRADS lexicon includes additional descriptors specific to ultrasound imaging, such as shape, orientation, margin, and echo pattern of lesions. These descriptors allow mammographers and radiologists to assess the likelihood of malignancy based on sonographic characteristics. For example, a lesion with irregular margins, posterior acoustic shadowing, and hypoechoic echotexture would raise suspicion for malignancy and be categorized accordingly [31].

The role of mammographers is critical in ensuring the accurate implementation of the BI-RADS and US-BIRADS lexicon [53]. Mammographers are responsible for acquiring high-quality images and working closely with radiologists to provide detailed descriptions of breast findings. Proper positioning, image optimization, and understanding the appropriate application of each BI-RADS category ensure that lesions are accurately classified, which directly impacts patient management. Their expertise contributes to reducing unnecessary biopsies for benign findings and ensuring timely interventions for suspicious abnormalities [53–55].

1.3 Special Imaging Modalities

After completing mammographic imaging, the next step typically involves B-mode ultrasound and/or elastography. Some departments have dedicated breast MRI facilities, which provide additional imaging support and enhance diagnostic accuracy. Moreover, contrast-enhanced mammography, tomosynthesis, and cone beam breast imaging are utilized to support clinical decision-making through various imaging methods.

1.3.1 Breast Ultrasound

B-mode ultrasound uses ultrasonic sound waves generated by a piezoelectric crystal and a mechanical oscillation process in the probe. These waves interact with, absorb, reflect, and attenuate various forms of energy as they pass through breast tissue. The returning echoes are received by the probe and converted into electrical signals, which are then used to produce the ultrasound image. Ultrasound is particularly advantageous in dense fibroglandular breast tissue, where mammogram sensitivity is reduced. It also offers features such as power Doppler, which can demonstrate hypervascularity around a region of interest and indicate the presence of a central feeding vessel in malignant findings [32, 33, 44, 56].

Ultrasound images of the breast occur due to the production of high-frequency sound waves which penetrate through soft tissue. As the sound waves pass through tissue, scattering, absorption, and reflection occur. Sound waves, which are bent by the incident tissue, spread with increasing depth, known as defocusing.

Ultrasound can delineate the skin, subcutaneous fat, breast parenchyma, retromammary fat, pectoralis muscle, ribs, and the anterior chest wall.

Various characteristics are used to distinguish benign and malignant lesions on ultrasound as seen in Table 1.3.

Patients with retro pectoral or prepectoral breast prosthesis benefit from the use of ultrasound as an adjunct method. If there is the suspicion of rupture or leakage, the ultrasound depicts a typical "snowstorm" appearance of the extravasated silicon contents into the surrounding tissue and axillary lymph nodes. The snowstorm appearance is due to inherent noise being produced from the silicone globules causing a delay in the sound waves being directed through breast tissue. The loss of coherence in the ultrasound waves is believed to cause the snowstorm of noise. A ruptured implant also has a similar MRI appearance of a "stepladder" along the folding of the implant surface, and it is also known as the "linguini sign" [57].

Over the years the contents and structure of implants have vastly improved with more patients opting for saline-type prosthesis, which has less risk of infection following rupture or extravasation. It is important to ask a patient for a mammogram what type of prosthesis was inserted and how long ago was the procedure performed, as this helps with the clinical assessment during imaging studies.

Intracapsular implant ruptures occur when the elastomer membrane of a silicone implant is still confined within the fibrous capsule surrounding the ruptured implant (see Fig. 1.21). Folds of the collapsing elastomer membrane are seen as thin, double

Table 1.3 Malignant, indeterminate, and benign characteristics [33]

Malignant	Indeterminate	Benign
Spiculation	Maximum diameter	Round, oval shaped
Angular margins	Isoechogenicity	Macro lobulations less than 3
Marked hypo echogenicity	Mild hypo echogenicity	Thin echogenic pseudocapsule
Shadowing	Enhanced posterior enhancement	Peripheral vascularity
Calcification	Heterogeneous internal echotexture	
Duct extension	Homogeneous internal echogenicity	
Branch pattern	Central vascularity or central feeding vessel	
Microlobulation		

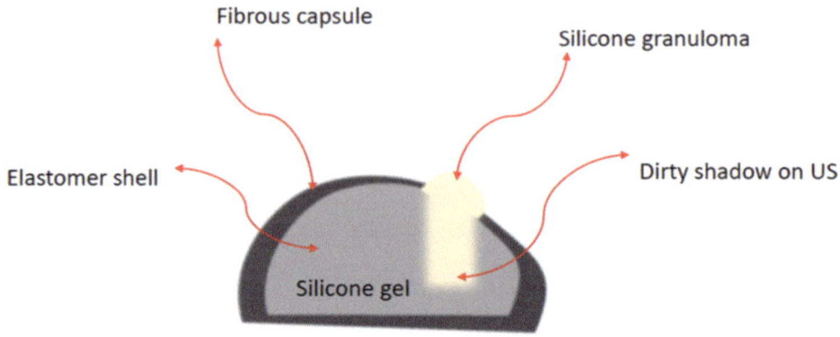

Fig. 1.21 Sonographic appearance of an intracapsular rupture

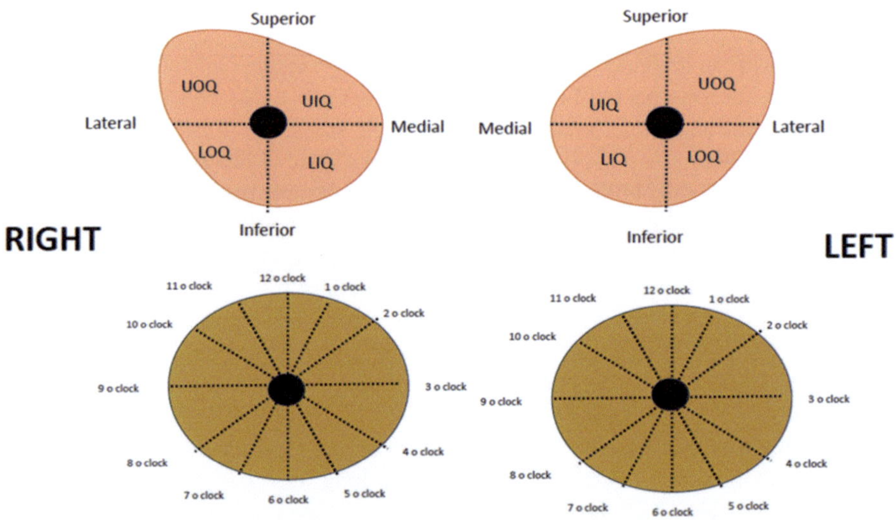

Fig. 1.22 Breast o clock system used for ultrasound reporting

echogenic lines called the "stepladder sign" in sonographic literature counterpart to the MRI finding called the "linguini sign."

Axial resolution: Is the visualization of structures parallel to the skin (such as mammary ducts) (see Fig. 1.22). It allows the identification of the capsule characteristics surrounding cysts and solid lesions. Lateral resolution: Is used to reduce volume averaging of surrounding normal breast tissues with pathological lesions. There are two planes which affect lateral resolution: the long axis and short axis [12, 25, 32, 33, 38, 44, 56, 58–61].

In general lateral resolution improves with increasing the number of channels, aperture size, the number of elements in the transducer, and scan lines. Electronic focusing on transmit depends on many of the same factors as receive focusing but is more limited. It depends upon the number of transmit zones. In general, the more transmit zones, the better the lateral resolution. However, increasing the number of transmit zones decreases the frame rate. In general, multiple transmit focal zones in the first 2 cm are very beneficial in breast sonography.

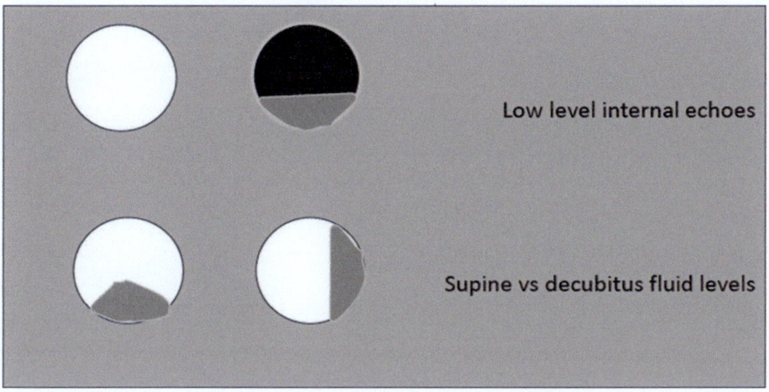

Fig. 1.23 Sonographic descriptions of fluid levels in cystic lesions

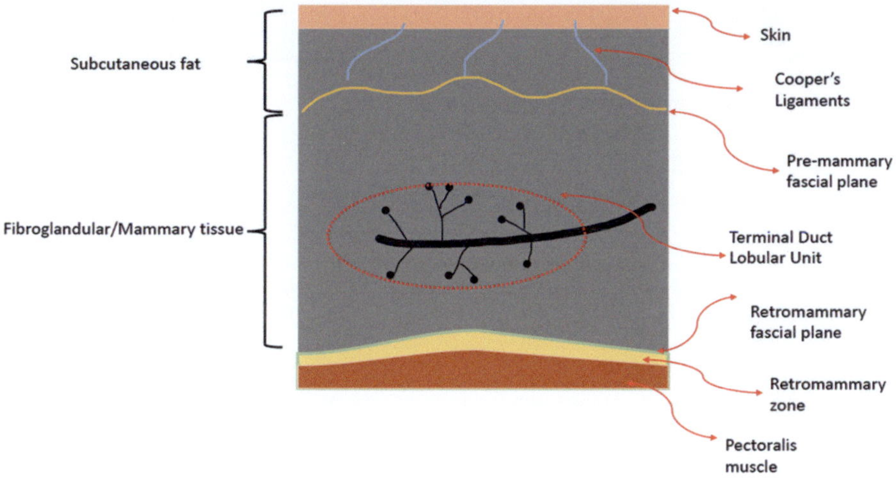

Fig. 1.24 Anatomical appearance of breast tissue on ultrasound

The measurement of a mass/cyst requires both a longitudinal and transverse measurement at 90-degree angle. Malignancy typically depicts as a "longer than tall" appearance, measuring over 1.4 for length/AP ratio (see Figs. 1.23, 1.24, and 1.25) [33, 44].

A. Zones of the breast.
B. Documentation of depth of tissue.
C. Localization of mass in the right breast.
D. Anterior and posterior mammogram of the breast.
E. Longitudinal view of the breast mass.
F. Medial to lateral mammogram acquisition.

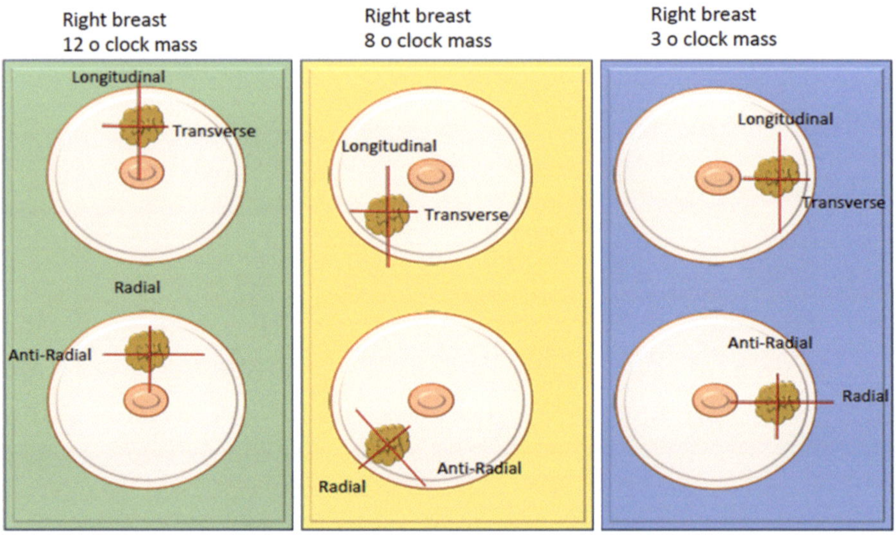

Fig. 1.25 Various scanning methods for breast masses

Fig. 1.26 How annotation of a breast mass occurs

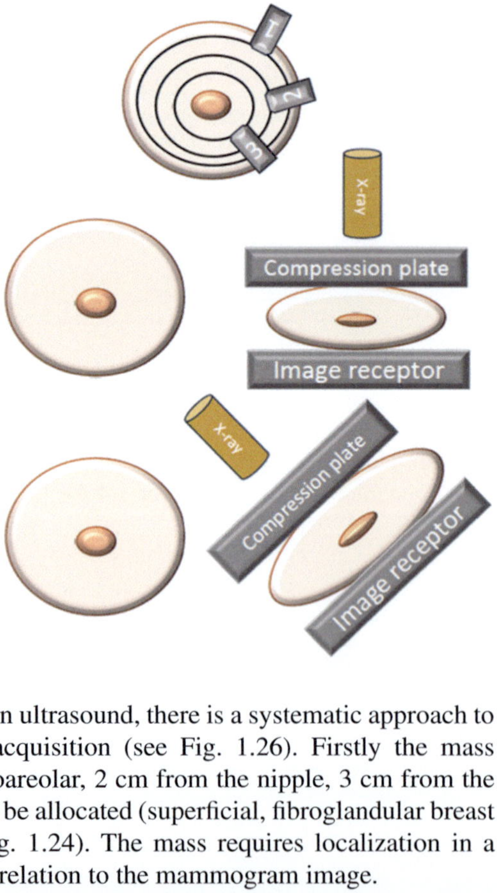

When a breast mass is annotated on ultrasound, there is a systematic approach to allow correlation to mammogram acquisition (see Fig. 1.26). Firstly the mass requires a zone of breast tissue (retroareolar, 2 cm from the nipple, 3 cm from the nipple). The depth of the tissue has to be allocated (superficial, fibroglandular breast tissue, retromammary space (see Fig. 1.24). The mass requires localization in a breast o'clock position as well as correlation to the mammogram image.

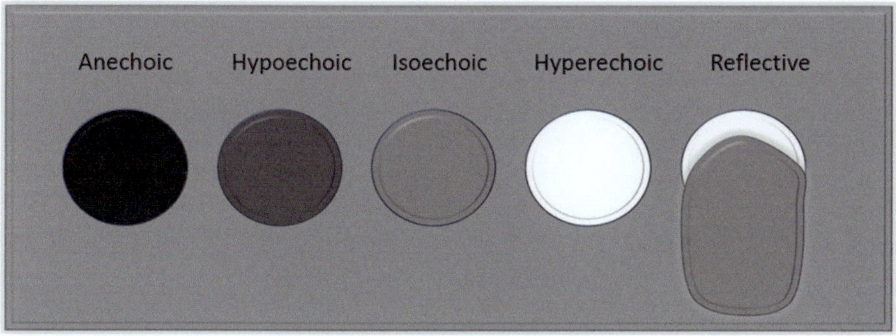

Fig. 1.27 Various levels of echogenicity on ultrasound

Depending on the attenuation characteristic of various tissues within the breast, the subsequent ultrasound image will result in various shades of gray (see Figs. 1.23 and 1.27). Cysts which consist of fluid content have an anechoic appearance with strong posterior acoustic enhancement, which relates to benign findings. Calcifications or bony structures do not allow follow-through of sound waves, producing a strong posterior hypoechoic shadow. Malignancy however can be depicted as both hyper- and hypoechoic in echogenicity.

Shear wave elastography [12] builds on the concept of palpating tissue with ultrasound waves, emitting lateral shear waves that provide information on the elasticity index of a visualized mass. This technique allows some systems to measure tissue density, offering a high predictive rate for positive diagnoses and histological outcomes. A Tsukuba score index tool was developed, as seen in Fig. 1.28 which provides a grading scale from benign to malignant findings:

Breast MRI is an additional tool (see Fig. 1.29) used to determine the extent of disease or confirm its presence when mammography or ultrasound findings are inconclusive. Contrast-enhanced mammography, using imaging methods similar to interventional radiology's image subtraction technique, has shown promise in detecting occult masses missed by standard imaging techniques [7, 33].

1.3.2 Contrast-Enhanced Digital Mammography (CEDM)

Involves the intravenous injection of iodinated contrast media along with mammographic evaluation. The two main types currently used are temporal subtraction and dual-energy technique. Temporal subtraction used high-energy digital mammography images and subtraction of pre-contract from post-contrast images (see Fig. 1.30) [23, 63].

Dual-energy technique (see Fig. 1.31) assesses the energy dependence of x-ray attenuation through materials of various densities, i.e., contrast and soft tissue. A pair of low- and high-energy images are produced post-contrast injection and are then combined to enhance regions of contrast uptake.

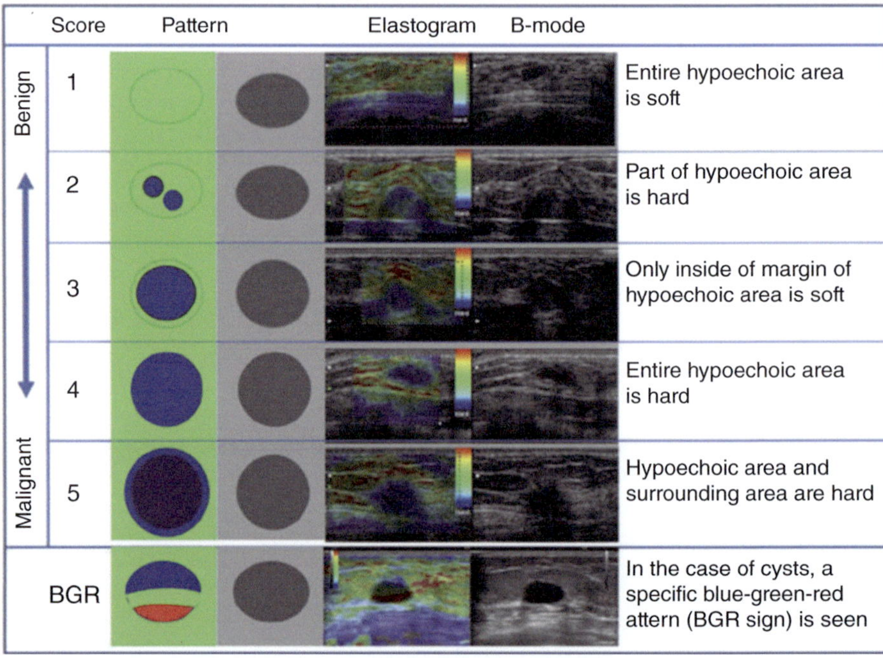

Fig. 1.28 Tsukuba score index [62]

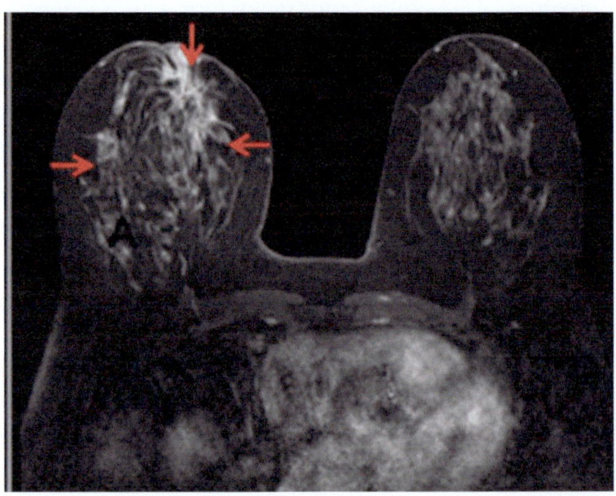

Fig. 1.29 Example of a multicentric malignancy visualized on the T1 weighted MRI image of the right breast [3]

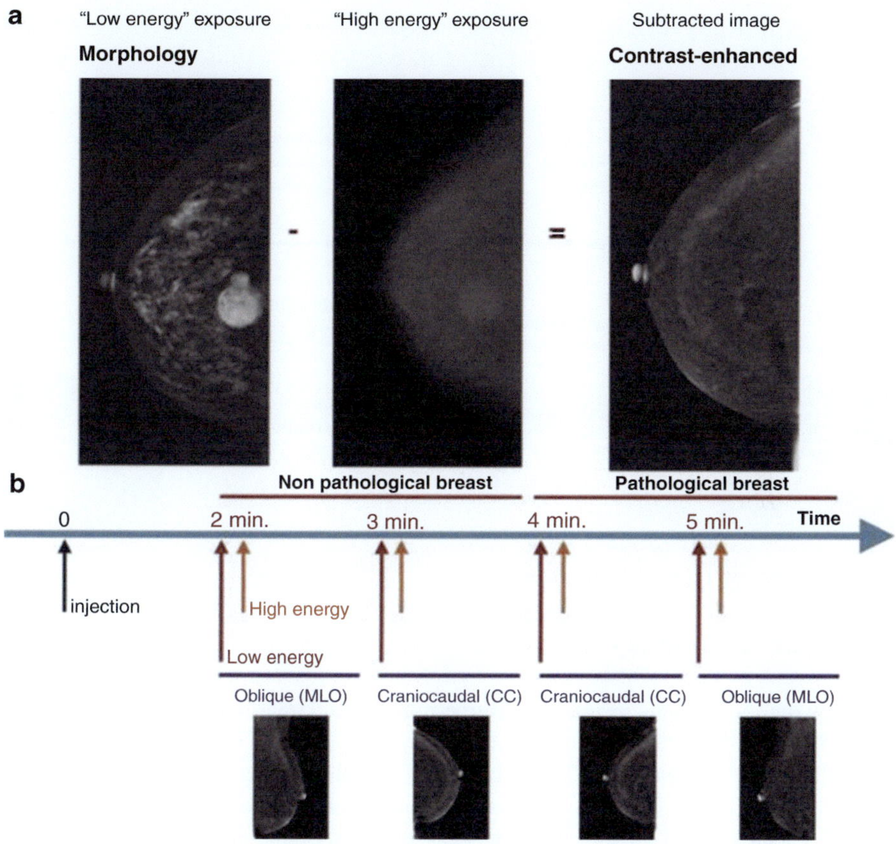

Fig. 1.30 Temporal subtraction contrast-enhanced digital mammography

The advantages of CEDM are that it is able to demonstrate neovascularity associated with malignancy and improves the malignancy detection rate.

The uses of CEDM are:

- Determining extent of disease.
- Assessment of recurrent disease.
- Clarification of unequivocal lesions.
- Detection of occult lesions with dense breast tissue.
- Monitoring the response to chemotherapy.
- Utilized as a staging tool.

The limitation of CEDM is the increased risk of false negative rate for nonvascular tumors such as lymphangitis carcinomatosis.

The future role of CEDM will be the joint use thereof with tomosynthesis technology.

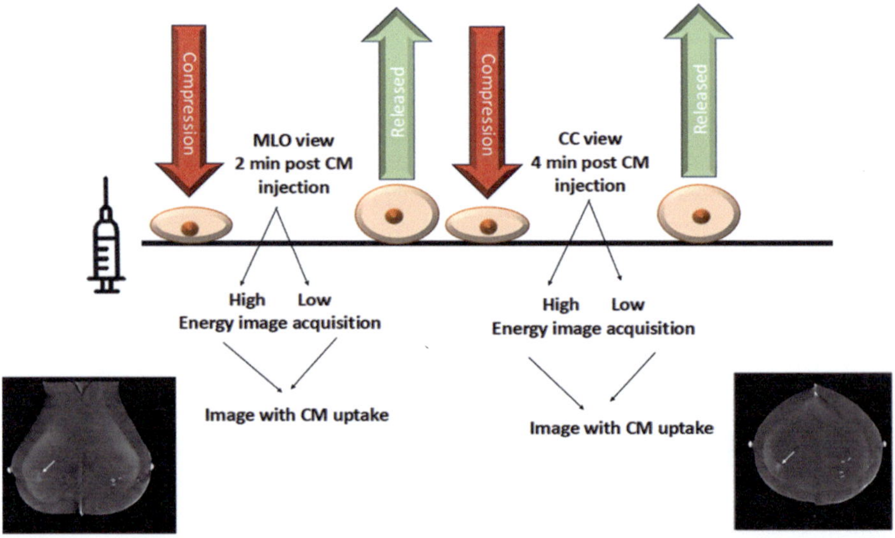

Fig. 1.31 Dual-energy CEDM technique

1.3.3 Breast Tomosynthesis

The new mammographic technique of three-dimensional imaging (digital breast tomosynthesis DBT or breast computed tomography CT) is based on the well-known concept of tomography (see Fig. 1.32). In breast CT, the breast hangs in a small gantry, like conventional CT scanners, and the breast is scanned as in incremental CT. With DBT, a smaller scan angle is utilized with the x-ray source moving around the breast within the range of the angle. The use of a smaller scan angle allows faster interpretation and acquisition of images. The main function of DBT is to visualize previously occult lesions, obscured by overlying soft tissue structures on 2D images [3, 4, 7, 64].

It is still being debated whether the leafing between a stack of images may impair detection of certain morphological discrepancies or whether it improves the radiologist's interpretation methodology (see Fig. 1.33). The standard rates of mean glandular dose rates with DBT and breast CT also need to be reevaluated since a variability of 5–13% in MGD has been reported.

1.3.4 Computerized Tomography Laser Mammography (CTLM)

Is an optical tomographic technique using laser energy (see Fig. 1.34) in the near infrared spectra for detection of angiogenesis and hemoglobin distribution of malignancy? A laser detector measures the intensity drop during attenuation through various breast tissue structures resulting in a tomography image [20].

The disadvantages of CTLM are the complexity and time cost of the procedure as well as poor interpretation outcomes due to human error rates and lack of appropriate CAD systems.

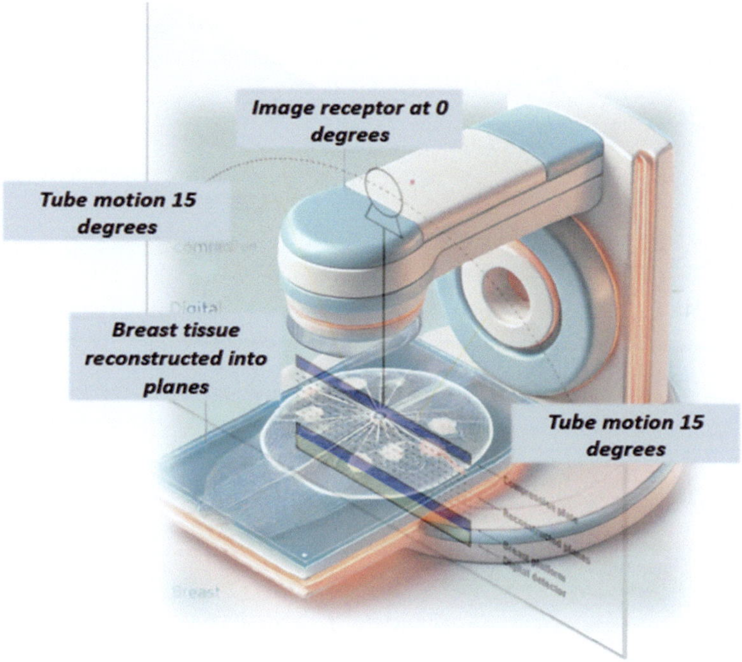

Fig. 1.32 Digital breast tomosynthesis

1.3.5 Positron Emission Mammography

Recently gained FDA approval to be used as adjunct to screening mammography and ultrasound techniques (see Figs. 1.35 and 1.36). It boasts a high resolution and localized region of interest. It uses dedicated gamma radiation detectors above and below the breast with mild breast compression applied. Fluorine-18 fluorodeoxy-glucose (18F-FDG) is administered to detect coincident gamma ray emission. The principle of the procedure lies in the basic physiology of a breast tumor which utilized glucose during cell metabolism. The increased use of glucose can be visualized through administration of 18F-FDG [15].

Indications

- When a mass is inconspicuous on mammogram and ultrasound.
- Patient with diffuse scattered breast calcifications.
- Where ultrasound was unable to delineate a mass in dense breast tissue.
- In altered post-radiation breast tissue.
- Lesions unable to be classified according to BI-RADS.
- When MRI of the breasts are contra-indicated.

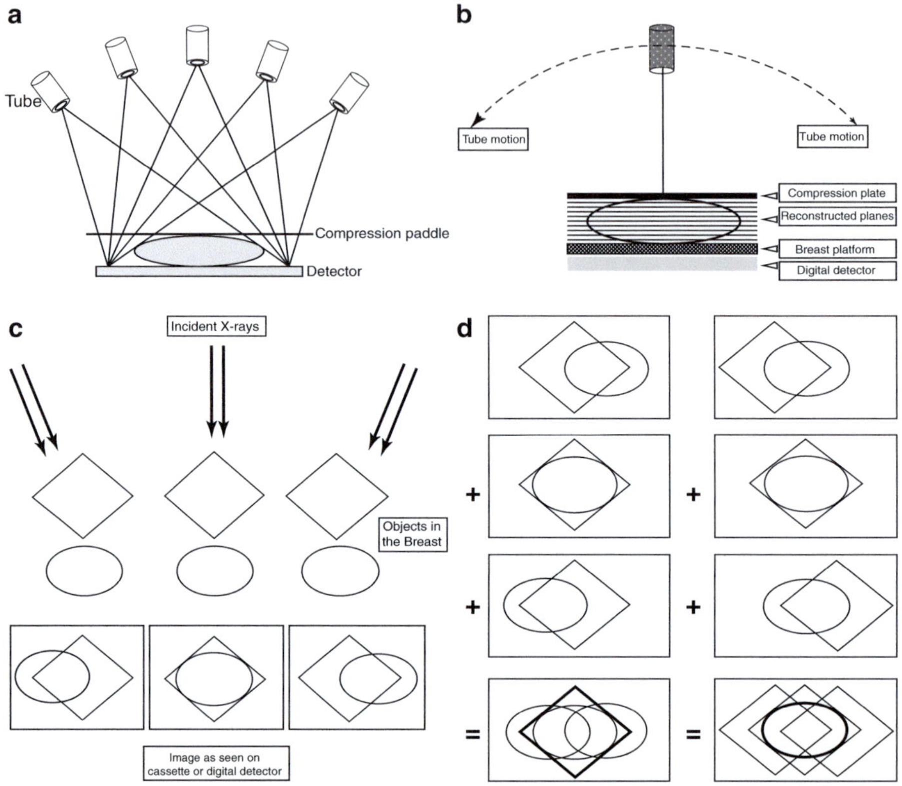

Fig. 1.33 Basic technologic principles of breast tomosynthesis [3, 4, 7, 64]. (**a**, **b**) Schemas show how image data are acquired from various angles as the x-ray tube moves in an arc. (**c**, **d**) Diagrams show how different 3D image data acquired from different angles (**c**) are reconstructed to provide separate depiction of two overlapping structures located in different planes (**d**)

Advantages	Disadvantages
Improved lesion delineation	Increased radiation exposure dose
Improved PPV	Not a screening method
Reduces workload	Low rate of repeatability
Tool for preoperative planning	
Good pathological correlation	
Effective for follow-up radiation therapy	

1.3.6 Automated Breast Ultrasound (ABUS)

Also known as 3D volume breast scanning is an ultrasound machine capable of scanning up to 350 images of the breast, which are then rendered into 3D format. It combines multiple ultrasound image frames, canceling out any random variation

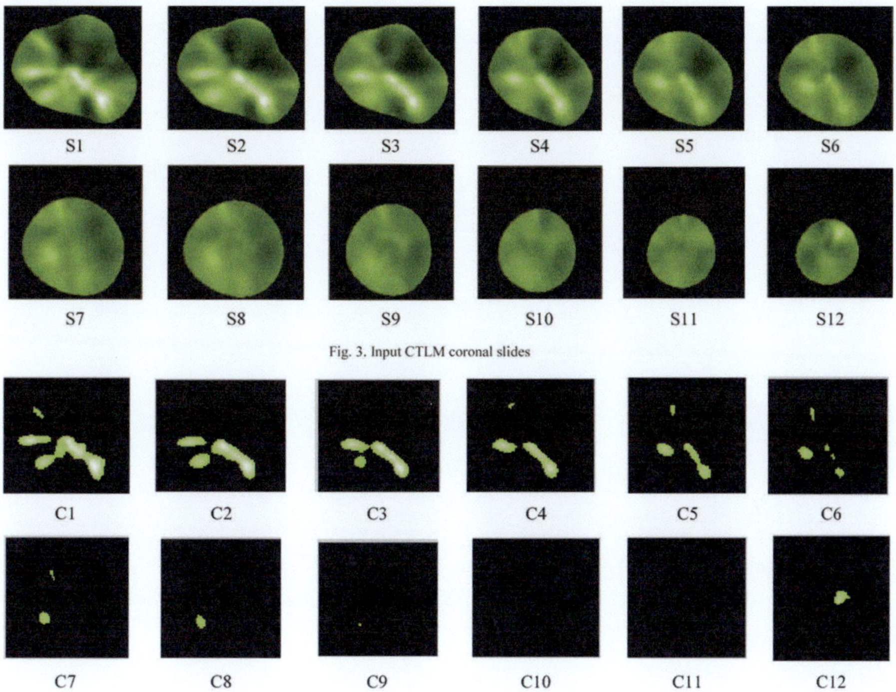

Fig. 1.34 CTLM image acquisition [20]

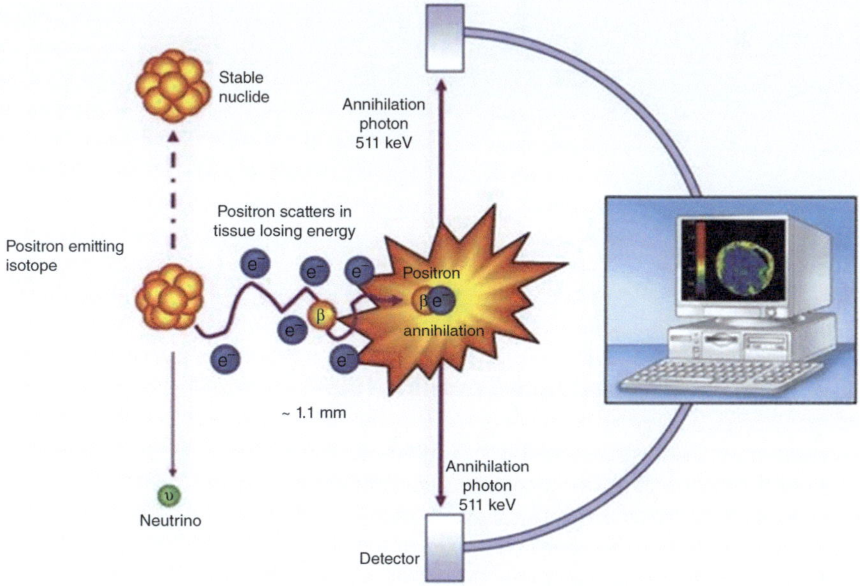

Fig. 1.35 Positron emission tomography principle [15]

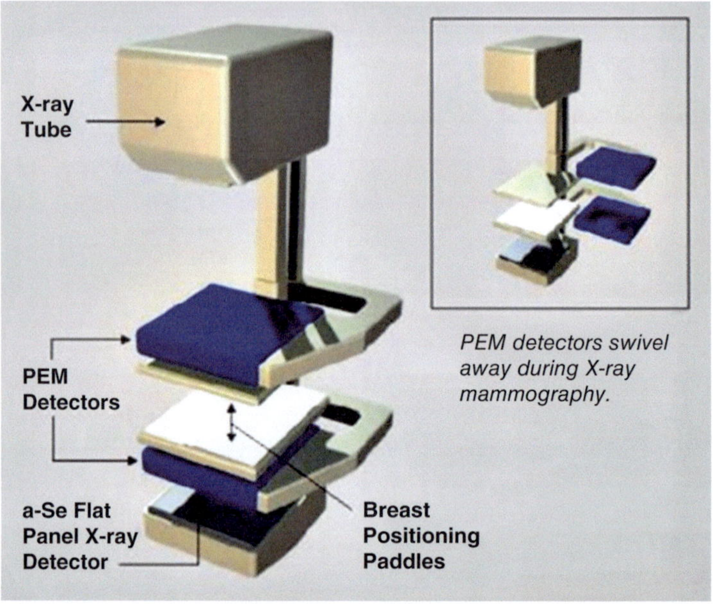

Fig. 1.36 PEM unit components [15]

(noise) which ultimately improves the signal-to-noise ratio. The procedure is well reproducible allowing comparison and follow-up imaging. Images are acquired in systematic longitudinal rows with overlapping of images to ensure complete analysis review.

Advantages	Disadvantages
Automated acquisition	Uses fixed width and depth settings
Wide field of view	Doppler and elastography not available during imaging
Rapid point of reference	Lymph node assessment is limited
Able to render coronal, sagittal, and transverse planes	Many imaging artifacts present: Skin folds Breathing

1.3.7 Electrical Impedance Scanning (EIS)

Also known as T-scan measures low-level bio-electric currents, producing real-time images of the electrical impedance properties of the breast (see Fig. 1.37). This delineates normal breast tissue from malignant changes. The T-scan (see Fig. 1.38) produces an image map of the breast by means of low electric current traversing through the breast and then measured at skin level with a probe on the skin surface [65].

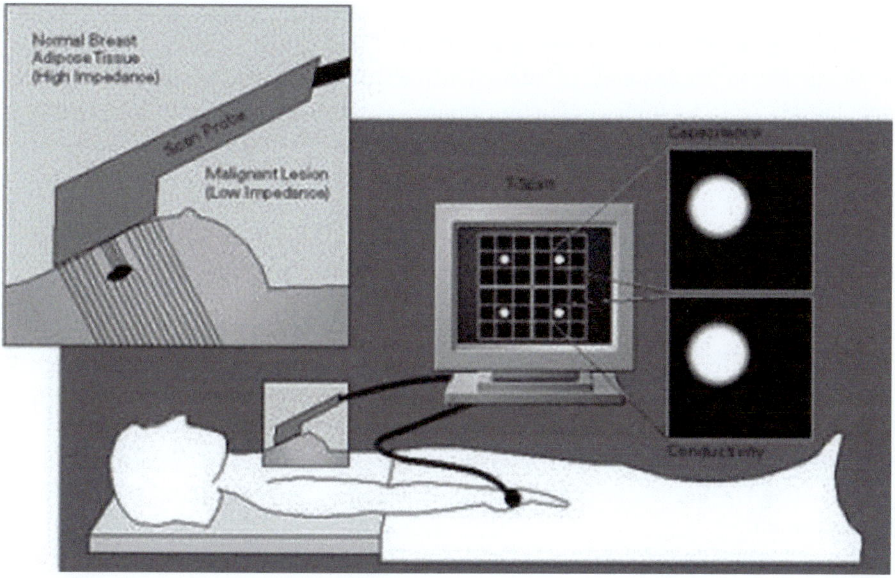

Fig. 1.37 Electrical impedance techniques [65]

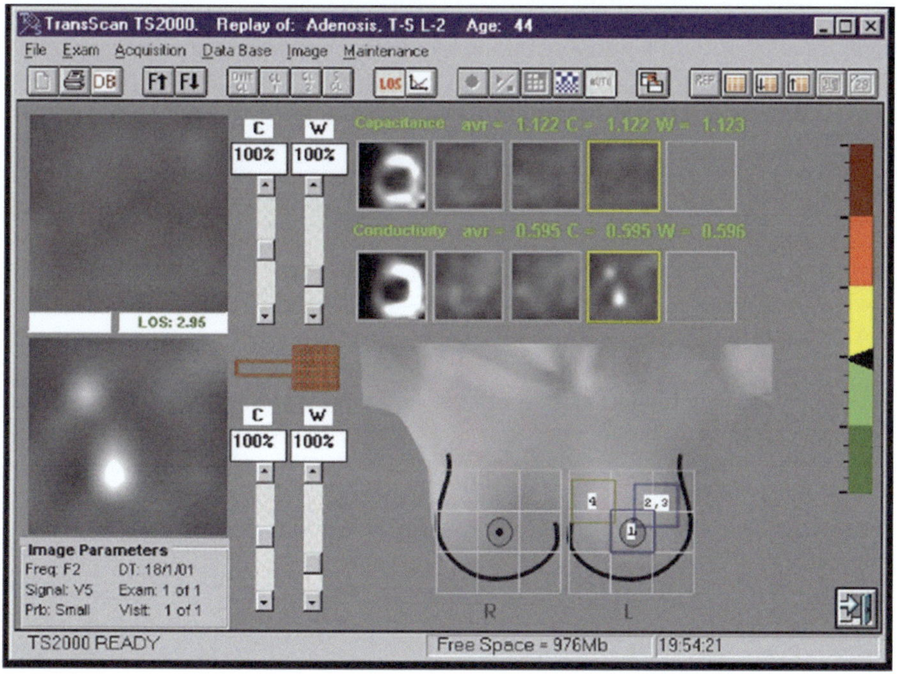

Fig. 1.38 Trans-scan interface display [65]

It uses no ionizing radiation, radionuclides, or breast compression technique [65].

There are many reported limitations to EIS such as the increased rate of false positives due to the presence of internal artifacts such as bone, muscle, and superficial lesions causing high-conduction images (bright spots). It also has a limited depth measured of up to 3.5 cm, thus excluding chest wall lesions. It is also not possible to localize a mass for biopsy [65].

1.3.8 Computer-Aided Detection, Artificial Intelligence (AI), and Deep Machine Learning (DML)

The biggest form of radiological technology advancement is the use of artificial intelligence and deep machine learning methods to decrease the rate of human detection errors from single reader analysis.

AmCAD Biomed based in Tokyo has developed multiple FDA-approved algorithms using DML to accurately differentiate between benign and malignant lesions on ultrasound.

Koios Medical has joined forces with GE Healthcare to develop a breast AI system for ultrasound capable of determining the BI-RADS rating of a mass using its morphological features and segmentation methods [20, 21, 42, 66–68].

The big question surrounding AI is the fear of machines taking over the role of the interpreter and technician. It is however well documented and explained by understanding AI will be used in radiology to augment the current service and not replace it.

AI is only as efficient as the training data fed to its DML system by a human. The cognitive skills and emotional role a physician has with their patient will not be easily reproduced by man-made machinery or AI systems.

Having said that, AI in radiology is an ever-expanding business and will most definitely disrupt the medical sector in the not-too-distant future [20, 21, 42, 66–68].

1.4 Image-Guided Biopsy

For many years, the initial method of diagnosing a mass was through direct surgical intervention. However, the common train of thought in the current medical era is that image-guided needle biopsy techniques are the best method for determining the type of breast lesion. The histology results may lead to the surgeon planning for a wider surgical excision, reducing the risk for a second operation due to positive margins [49].

1.4.1 Fine Needle Aspiration

Fine needle aspiration involves the placement of a 23–25-gauge needle into a mass to aspirate cells for further cytological assessment. The aspirated cells can be smeared onto a cytological slide and are then fixed with cytological fixing spray for immediate interpretation and diagnosis by the pathologist.

Advantages of FNA include:

- Cyto-pathologists opt for conservative reports, thus reducing the false-positive rates.
- There is a risk of sampling error (missing the actual mass).
- Less trauma and anxiety associated with FNA procedure for the patient.

Disadvantages of FNA:

- Operator dependent for both performing and interpreting the FNA.
- Vigor of oscillating the needle in target tissue depends on the FNA accuracy result.
- Limited to distinguishing benign from malignant cells, cannot differentiate types [49].

1.4.2 Core Needle Biopsy

Core needle biopsy (CNB) involves the removal of intact pieces of breast tissue (called specimens) which allows histological analysis. The biopsy is obtained through large gauge needles (11–18 size gauge). The removal of sample tissue is performed under local anesthetic through small 1–2 mm skin incisions.

Advantages of CNB:

- Tissue is prepared in formalin as with surgical excision which allows easy analysis by the pathologist.
- Less trauma for patients as with surgical excision, as no sutures are required.
- More cost effective than surgical intervention.

Disadvantage of CNB:

- Risk of sampling error especially with spring-driven biopsy needles.
- Large gauge needles increase the risk of hematoma/bleeding/infection [49].

Concordance between histological and radiologic findings is very important during the clinical assessment process:

If a mass was round, well-defined, and the histology proves a fibroadenoma, there is concordance between the two measuring methods.

If only a few calcifications were removed during the biopsy and the result is benign, the physician should not rely on the biopsy results alone for further clinical work up.

A radial scar with any atypical hyperplasia within the pathology report should be referred for further surgical intervention [49].

1.4.3 Localization

Localization is used for nonpalpable masses to guide the surgeon's approach to removal of a suspicious mass. It is safe and accurate and allows minimal invasive approach to surgical incision. The stereotactic approach will always be for the shortest route to the region of interest by using a 3D approach to the x,y,z coordinates/ parameters. During the localization procedure the radiologist must be confident of the lesion's location on both CC and MLO projections.

Localization needles include a simple hypodermic needle with a hook wire within its core (see Fig. 1.39). The purpose of the hook wire is to enter through the mass and with expulsion of the hypodermic/introductory needle, hook into the breast tissue to ensure stability and accuracy with subsequent surgical removal. Common items included with this procedure are local anesthetic (10 mg/mL), cleaning solution (chlorhexidine in water), syringe with 25 G needle, and a localization wire needle. Depending on the lesion span, the localization can either be single wire, for masses less than 2 cm and within one breast quadrant, or can be multiple wires, referred to as bracketing if it is multifocal, larger than 2 cm and in more than one quadrant of the breast [49].

Before the biopsy or localization can occur, the selection of the correct image modality needs to occur. The mass with architectural distortion is best served with ultrasound, whereas a mass with calcifications extending beyond the border of the mass is best utilized with mammography. Focal asymmetry without ultrasound correlate or post-biopsy clip imaging is also best seen with mammography (see Fig. 1.40). Larger lesions can also be bracketed to define the total volume for the surgeon [49].

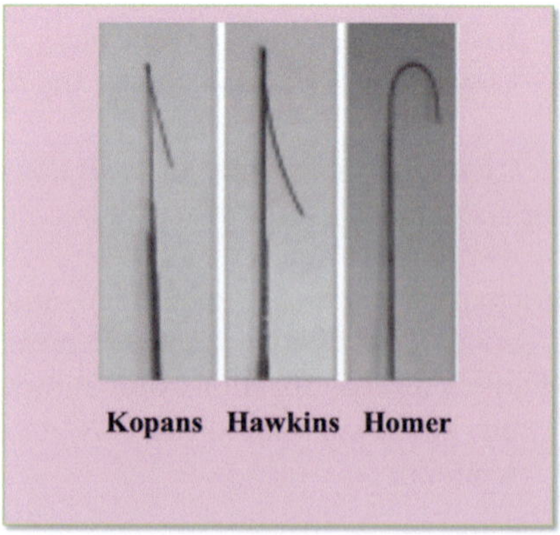

Fig. 1.39 Three most common types of localization needles used

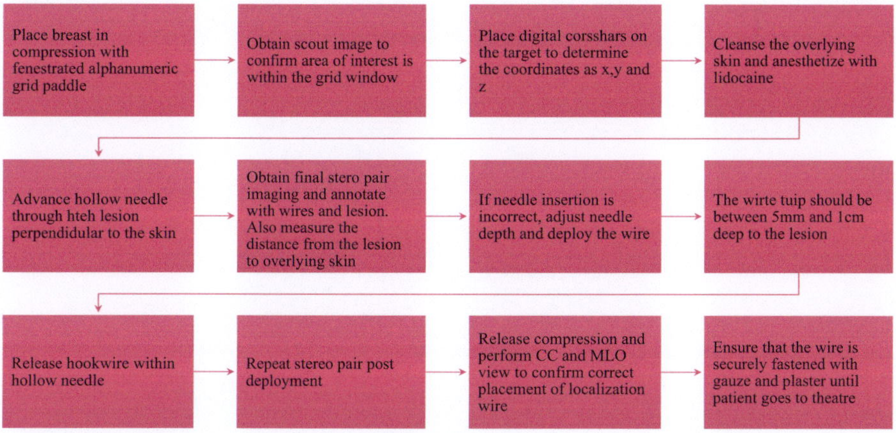

Fig. 1.40 Mammographic needle localization

> **Trick of the Trade**
> The needle wire has cm markings on the outer surface to aid in-depth placement.

The stepwise process for mammography needle-guided localization is seen below in Fig. 1.40.

1.4.4 Galactogram

Also known as a ductogram or contrast-assisted mammogram outlines the ductal system to provide information on nipple discharges and their origin site. It is indicated for patients with unilateral or spontaneous discharge with a bloody/clear appearance (see Fig. 1.41).

Ductogram kits contain a small gauge cannula which can be either straight or curved tip 30 gauge.

Other equipment includes:

- Non-ionic contrast media.
- Small 5 cc syringe.
- 19 gauge needles to contrast extraction
- Cytology slides.
- Fixative spray.
- Tape.
- Magnifying glasses.
- Bright light for introduction of needle into duct orifice.
- Nursing pad is used for post-procedure [49]

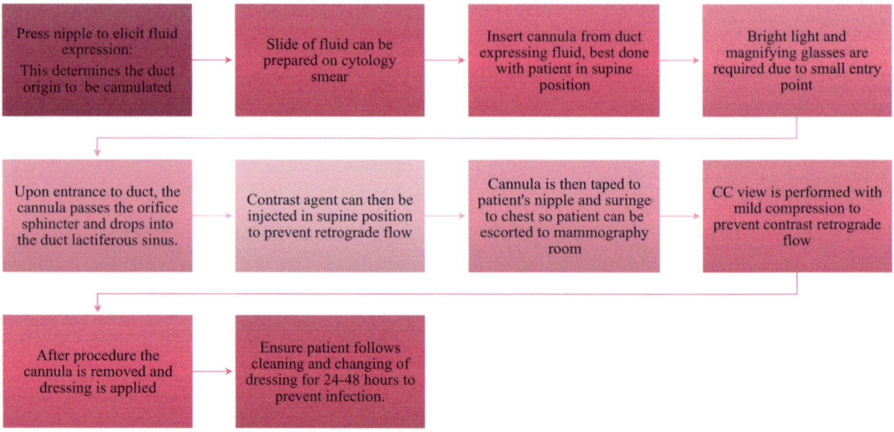

Fig. 1.41 Mammographic procedure for a galactogram

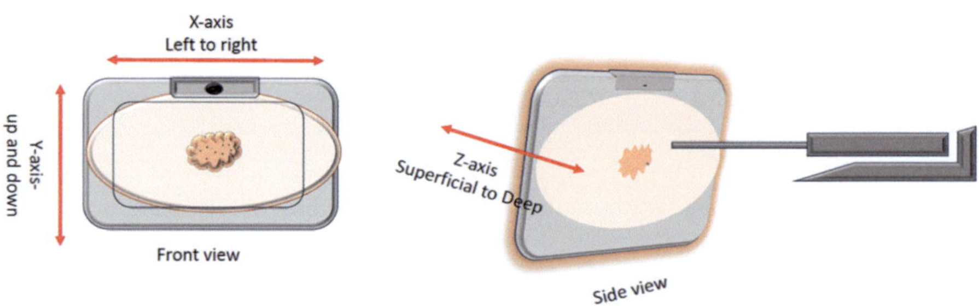

Fig. 1.42 Cartesian coordinate system

1.4.5 Stereotactic Mammography

Stereology is the science of determining 3D information of an object based on 2D (planar) views. The use of the stereotactic images, simple geometry, and 3D location of the lesion allows a mathematical calculation which can be used to accurately guide the needle into the lesion.

A stereotactic process consists of:

- *Stereo pair:* Two planar images of the abnormality at a 15-degree angle to each other (see Figs. 1.42, 1.43, and 1.44).
- *Reference point:* Providing the relative shift from the two stereo pair images to determine the x, y, and z coordinates.
- *Cartesian coordinates:* A cartesian system identifies the location of a unique point by three axes intersecting at right angles. For example: X = +4 mm, Y = 10 mm and Z = 22 m. The use of the system is important during troubleshooting of a stereotactic procedure. If the needle is 5 mm too far to the left of

Fig. 1.43 Stereotactic pair

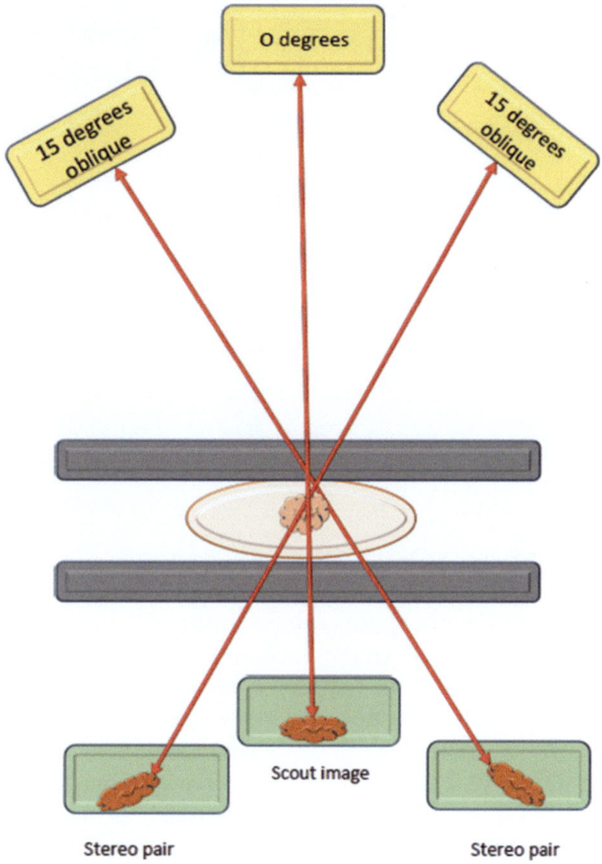

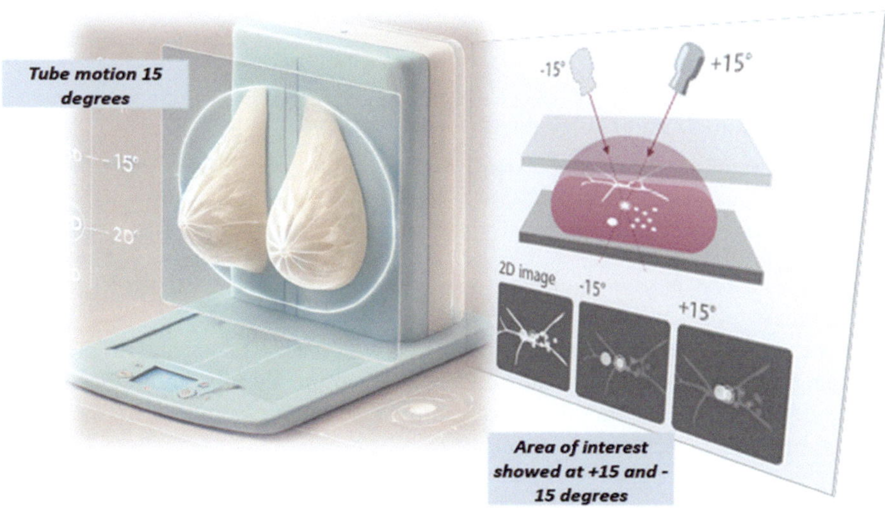

Fig. 1.44 Diagram representation of lesion as depicted by stereo pair

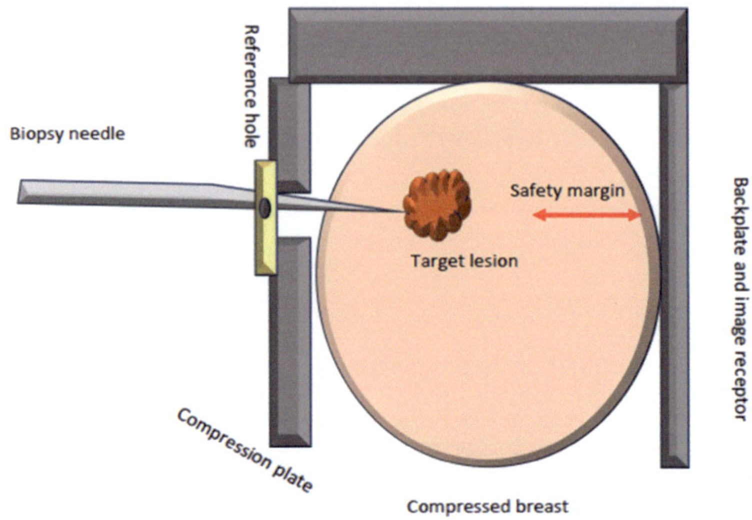

Fig. 1.45 Pre- and postfire images of stroke margin

the lesion, the needle can be corrected 5 mm to the right to ensure an accurate biopsy specimen representation (see Fig. 1.42).

- *Scout image* is the first step in obtaining the stereo pair. The x-ray tube is placed perpendicular to the breast tissue. The scout image is not used to obtain the localization coordinates. It facilitates as a reference image during the biopsy process.
- *Direction of shift:* With each stereo pair image, the projected abnormality will shift in the horizontal plane relative to its original position on the scout image (see Fig. 1.26).
- *Stroke margin* is the distance from the postfire position of the needle tip to the breast support, usually around 4 mm to allow a safe margin or stroke margin (see Fig. 1.45) [49].

> Stroke margin for proximal aspect of compressed breast = (compression thickness – 4/5 mm)—(prefire depth + stroke).
>
> Stroke margin for distal aspect of compressed breast = (prefire depth—stroke)—4/5 mm.

- *Positive stroke margin* indicates ample thickness for the needle to traverse the breast.
- *Negative stroke margin* indicates the needle will exit the breast and hit the backplate of system. To prevent a negative stroke margin, alter the prefire position of the needle tip, use a shorter stroke biopsy instrument, or reposition the breast (see Fig. 1.29).

- *Prefire back off:* is the position of the biopsy instrument which will place the center of the abnormality in the center of the sample notch allowing maximum capture of lesion (see Figs. 1.46 and Fig. 1.47) [49].

Preplanning procedure:

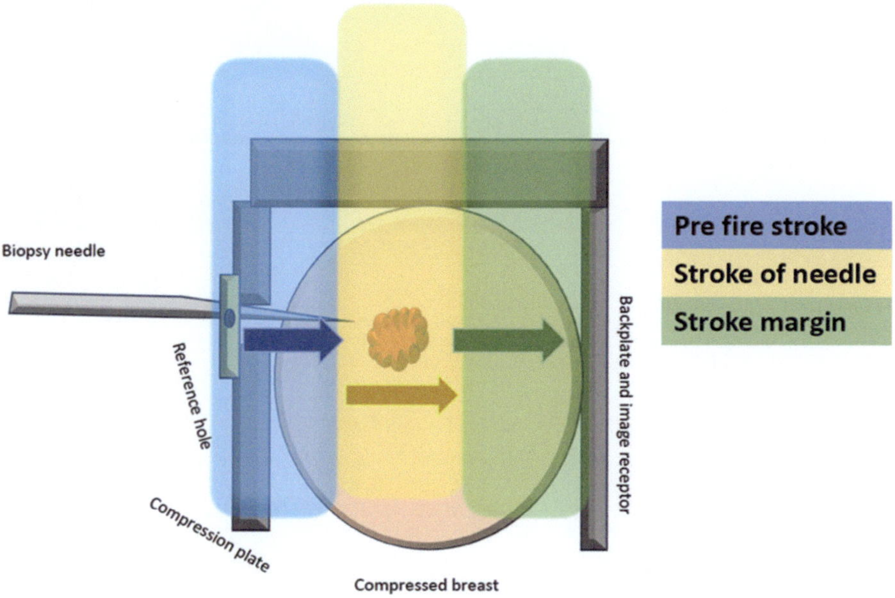

Fig. 1.46 Stroke margin principles

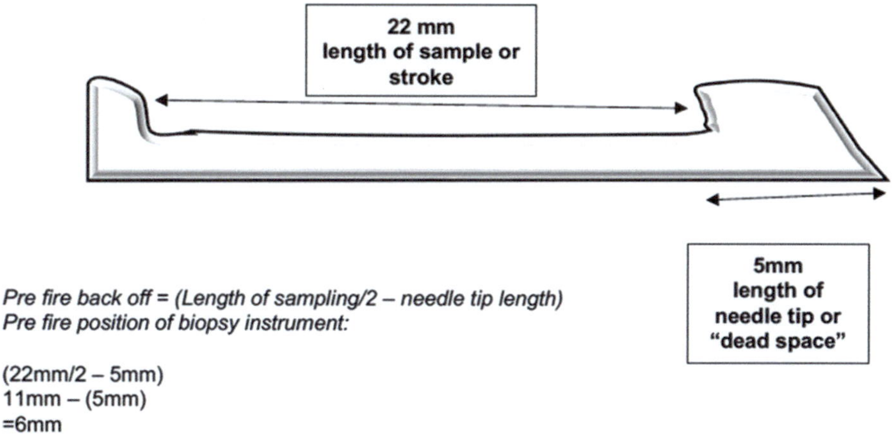

Fig. 1.47 Dead space of a needle

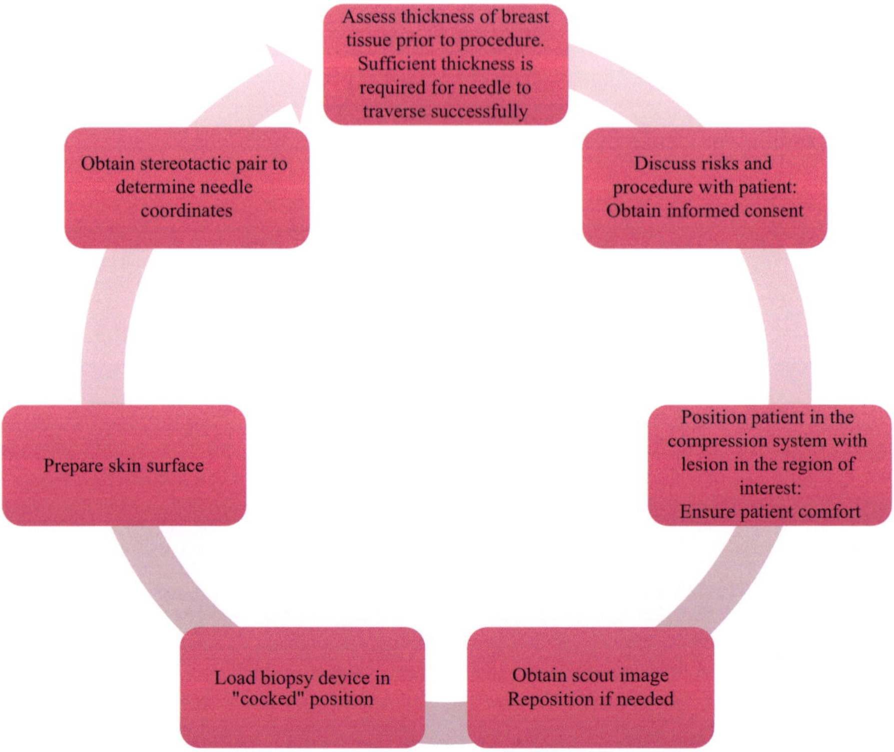

During procedure:

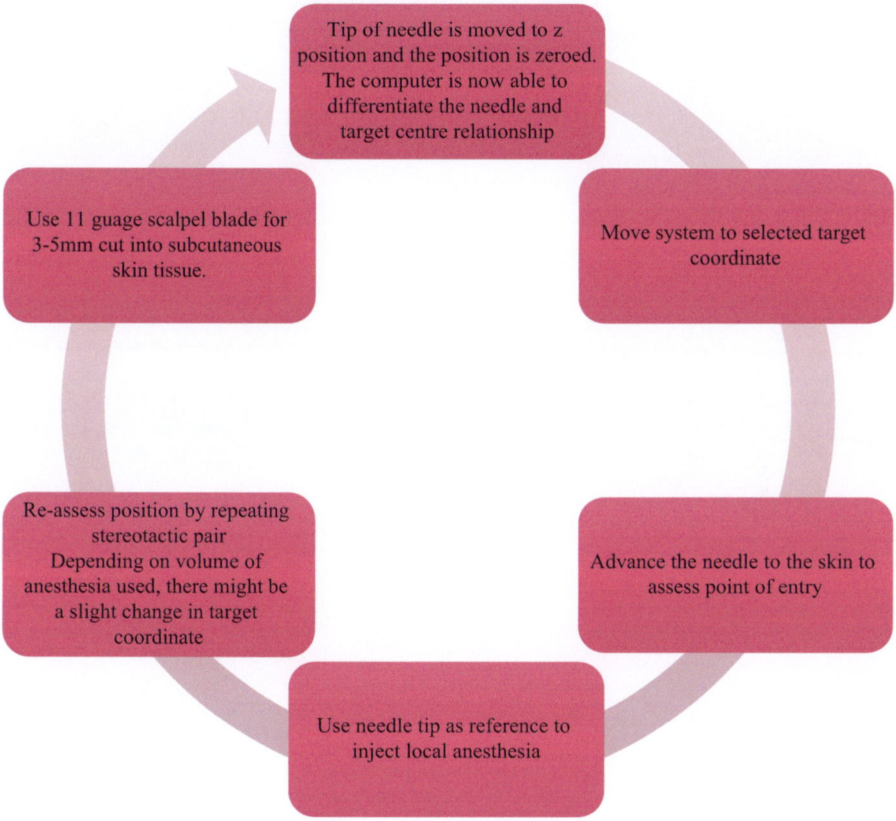

Stereotactic process:

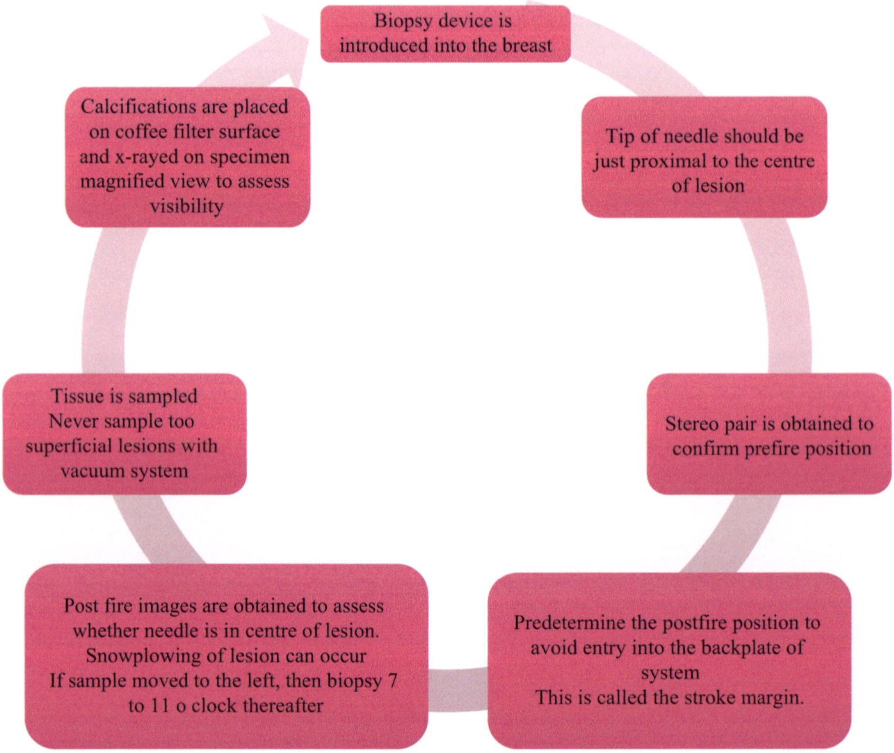

Post procedure:

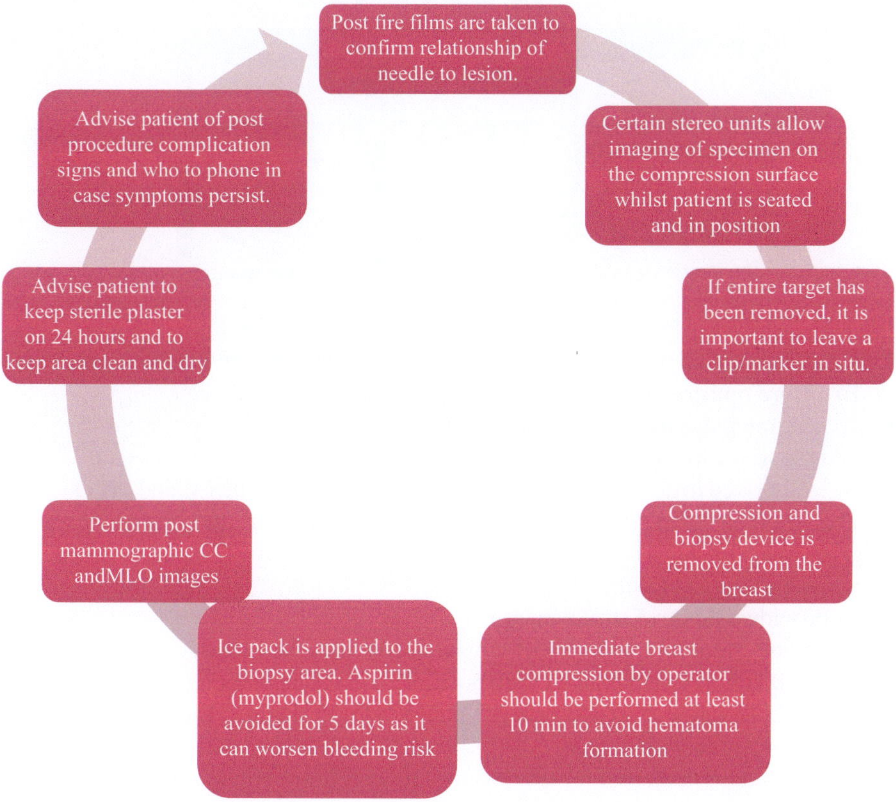

Troubleshooting for stereotactic procedures	
Breast is too thin	Can use posterior bolsters such as foam or towels to allow breast thickness to increase or use saline drip bag
Lesion to close to chest wall	On prone bed, bring patient's arm and shoulder through the stereo hole on table to allow visualization of deeper structures
Needle is in but lesion is too far to reach	Retract the needle tip, retarget the lesion, and reposition needle through same skin incision to avoid another entry site
Lesion not visible on stereo pair images	Some systems allow to use the scout and one stereo 15-degree image as a pair for depth measurement
Patient used aspirin, ibuprofen, or warfarin prior to procedure	Reschedule with 5–7 days of halting medication to avoid bleeding risk
Sampling error occurred	Patient may have moved during procedure; lesion may be of a dense consistency and difficult to penetrate. A 5 mm error in coordinates can also cause this.
Pathology report is discordant to radiologist report	Ensure than at least 5–7 biopsy specimens are taken during the procedure. Perform stereo targets around the lesion border and deeper to the lesion depth to ensure a true representative region of interest for pathology interpretation.

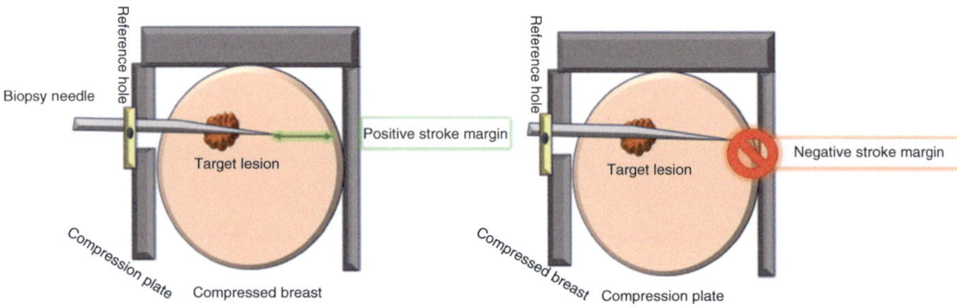

Fig. 1.48 Positive and negative stroke margin

- To ensure optimal patient comfort.
- To be knowledgeable of the stereotactic unit.
- Be able to grasp the concepts of stroke and stroke margin calculations.
- Be well versed in determining a lesion's position based on the CC and MLO views.
- The shortest skin to abnormality distance based on the initial mammogram images:
  - Will minimize trauma to the breast.
  - Provide a positive stroke margin.
  - Ensure minimal traversing of biopsy needle into the breast.
  - Ex: If lesion is at 12:00 o clock position, use CC approach.
  - Ex: If lesion is at 10:00 of right breast, use 45 degrees use superior-lateral, inferior-medial approach.
- Ensure patient cooperation with positioning and immobilization techniques.

When imaging indicates the need for further intervention, an image-guided biopsy is required. Ultrasound-guided biopsy is preferred for both patient comfort and ease of use by the referring specialist. Vacuum-assisted biopsy needles are used to retrieve large specimens during the procedure, ensuring that well-represented samples are sent to the histopathologist for assessment.

Stereotactic-guided biopsy is used for microcalcifications present in the breast, and in some instances for a vague density not well visualized on ultrasound. To ensure the correct area of interest is targeted during the biopsy, it is advised to make use of a CC and ML view prior to the procedure and to mark on the skin surface the target area during the biopsy [69].

During stereotactic-guided biopsy, there are many mathematical equations to be used to ensure that a successful biopsy is done. The first step is to have a good understanding of the biopsy needles used in your department, as the needle sampling area, dead space, may differ in length, between manufacturing vendors.

The dead space of a standard needle tip ranges from 5 to 8 mm, while the active sampling area typically measures 15–22 mm, and the active throw of the needle is usually 20–25 mm. Understanding the dead space is crucial as it is not used for sampling the region of interest; it merely serves as an entry point for the active sampling area to reach the target site.

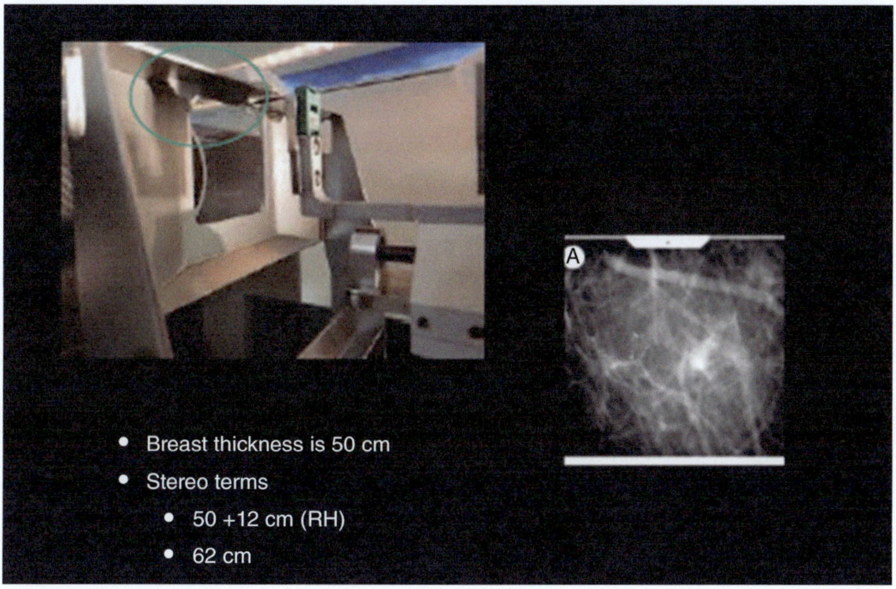

Fig. 1.49 Reference hole

The stereotactic system provides X, Y, and Z coordinates for any region marked during imaging, offering a 3D representation of the lesion's position left to right (X axis), up or down (Y axis), and depth (Z axis) within the breast.

Before planning a stereotactic biopsy, the breast density and placement of the region of interest (ROI) must be assessed to ensure the needle can enter without hitting the backplate of the mammogram machine.

A standard value added to the breast thickness indicated by the stereo unit is 12 mm, as this represents the reference hole (see Fig. 1.49) used during QC and zero-target setting of the system [69].

For instance, if the breast density is 30 mm and the mass is at a depth of 20 mm with a needle throw of 20 mm, the calculation is as follows:

1.5 Conclusion

In this chapter, we explored the diverse imaging modalities and techniques involved in diagnosing and understanding breast pathology, from foundational physics to advanced technological innovations. Starting with the physics underlying mammography, we reviewed both conventional and digital mammography, delving into the properties of digital images and various system types that enhance breast imaging quality and accuracy. The section on image interpretation highlighted the critical role of mammography in screening and diagnostics, including the interpretation

Stereo Test

Breast thickness measures as 30 mm, and thus automatically add 12 mm (for the reference hole which is considered a standard measure of thickness from the Z = 0 point).

30 + 12 = 42 mm.

Lesion Z measures at = 20 mm for the target.

If the needle tip starts at 20 mm, and it then "shoots" out another 20 mm (needle throw), the postfire position of the needle tip will be at 40 mm.

The total breast thickness is 42 mm, and the needle tip is at 40 mm when it has fired, and this only leaves a 2 mm margin of error and is not enough to be considered safe (need at least 4 mm safety margin).

To avoid this, the mammographer can adjust the angle of the breast tissue, use a sterile saline bag behind the breast, or change the needle's entry point.

In another example, if the breast tissue measures 50 mm, the scenario would be safe, as there would be **8** mm of tissue remaining after the needle is fired, avoiding the backplate.

Prefire Stereo Test

Following the pre-stereo test, the caliper targets the ROI. For instance, if the mass is set at:

X = 10 mm.
Y = 5 mm.
Z = 20 mm.

With a breast thickness of 65 mm, the needle tip is inserted just in front of the ROI at a caliper measure of:

X = 10 mm.
Y = 5 mm.
Z = 15 mm.

The needle has a throw of 20 mm, a dead space of 5 mm, and an active sampling area of 20 mm. Therefore:

Total breast thickness including reference hole is 65+ 12 mm = 72 mm.

15 mm (needle tip) + 20 mm throw = 35 mm end point postfire
35–5 mm (dead space) = 30 mm
30–20 mm (active sampling length) = 10 mm.

Thus, the needle will actively sample from 10 mm to 30 mm, encompassing the ROI at 20 mm, ensuring it is well placed within the active sampling portion of the needle.

Post-stereo Test

The same calculations apply post-biopsy to ensure the needle has not deviated from the X, Y, or Z axis during firing, as some lesions may be hard and difficult to penetrate with the biopsy needle. If a variance of more than 2 mm is noted, manual adjustment of the needle using the system's X, Y, and Z settings can realign it with the ROI caliper target measure.

It is advisable to print a post-biopsy image of any calcifications observed during stereotactic-guided biopsy imaging and attach it to the pathology referral note. This ensures that the histopathologist is aware of the presence of fine microcalcifications in the samples and can perform fine cuts of the frozen specimens for detailed analysis.

of calcifications, breast appearance variations, and unique considerations for male breast imaging, all contextualized within the BIRADS and US-BIRADS lexicon.

A comprehensive look at special imaging modalities underscored the evolving landscape of breast imaging, covering ultrasound, contrast-enhanced mammography, tomosynthesis, and more advanced tools like PET mammography, automated ultrasound, and electrical impulse scanning. Furthermore, we addressed the integration of computer-aided detection, artificial intelligence, and deep learning, which are transforming image analysis and aiding radiologists in achieving more precise diagnostics.

We also looked at the examination of image-guided biopsy techniques, including fine needle aspiration, core needle biopsy, and localization methods like stereotactic biopsy, each serving a critical function in accurately diagnosing breast pathology.

References

1. Hogg P, Kelly J, Mercer C. Digital mammography: a holistic approach. London: Springer; 2022.
2. Berg WA, Gutierrez L, NessAiver MS, Carter WB, Bhargavan M, Lewis RS, et al. Diagnostic accuracy of mammography, clinical examination, US, and MR imaging in preoperative assessment of breast cancer. Radiology. 2004;233(3):830–49.
3. Monticciolo DL, Newell MS, Moy L, Niell B, Monsees B, Sickles EA. Breast cancer screening in women at higher-than-average risk: recommendations from the ACR. J Am Coll Radiol. 2018;15(3 Pt A):408–14.
4. Tagliafico AS, Calabrese M, Mariscotti G, Durando M, Tosto S, Monetti F, et al. Adjunct screening with Tomosynthesis or ultrasound in women with mammography-negative dense breasts: interim report of a prospective comparative trial. J Clin Oncol. 2016;34(16):1882–8.
5. Berg WA, Leung K. In: Hooley D, Davis E, editors. Diagnostic imaging: breast. 3rd ed. Philadelphia: Elsevier; 2019.
6. Da Costa D, Taddese A, Cure ML, Gerson D, Poppiti R Jr, Esserman LE. Common and unusual diseases of the nipple-areolar complex. Radiographics. 2007;27(Suppl 1):S65–77.
7. Siu AL, Force USPST. Screening for breast cancer: U.S. preventive services task force recommendation statement. Ann Intern Med. 2016;164(4):279–96.

8. Barkana BD, El-Sayed A, Khaled RH, Helal M, Khaled H, Deeb R, et al. Imaging modalities in inflammatory breast cancer (IBC) diagnosis: a computer-aided diagnosis system using bilateral mammography images. Sensors (Basel). 2022;23(1)
9. Glassman LM. Pathology of the male breast; 2014
10. Cserni G, Francz M, Jaray B, Kalman E, Kovacs I, Krenacs T, et al. Pathological diagnosis, work-up and reporting of breast cancer 1st central-eastern European professional consensus statement on breast cancer. Pathol Oncol Res. 2022;28:1610373.
11. Mercer PHJKC. Digital mammography: a holistic approach. Springer Publisher; 2015.
12. Sigrist RMS, Liau J, Kaffas AE, Chammas MC, Willmann JK. Ultrasound Elastography: review of techniques and clinical applications. Theranostics. 2017;7(5):1303–29.
13. Miao YR, Zhang Q, Lei Q, Luo M, Xie GY, Wang H, et al. ImmuCellAI: a unique method for comprehensive T-cell subsets abundance prediction and its application in cancer immunotherapy. Adv Sci (Weinh). 2020;7(7):1902880.
14. Zhao W, Hunt DC, Tanioka K, Rowlands JA. Amorphous selenium flat panel detectors for medical applications. Nucl Instrum Methods Phys Res, Sect A. 2005;549(1–3):205–9.
15. Reznik A, Lui BJ, Rowlands JA. An amorphous selenium based positron emission mammography camera with avalanche gain. Technol Cancer Res Treat. 2005;4(1):61–7.
16. van Rooyen M, Becker T, Westraadt J, Marx G. Creep damage assessment of ex-service 12% Cr power plant steel using digital image correlation and quantitative microstructural evaluation. Materials (Basel). 2019;12(19)
17. Black E, Richmond R. Improving early detection of breast cancer in sub-Saharan Africa: why mammography may not be the way forward. Glob Health. 2019;15(1):3.
18. Thompson A, Brennan K, Cox A, Gee J, Harcourt D, Harris A, et al. Evaluation of the current knowledge limitations in breast cancer research: a gap analysis. Breast Cancer Res. 2008;10(2):R26.
19. Fico N, Di Grezia G, Cuccurullo V, Salvia AAH, Iacomino A, Sciarra A, Gatta G. Breast imaging physics in mammography (part I). Diagnostics. 2023;13(20):3227.
20. Jalalian A, Mashohor S, Mahmud R, Karasfi B, Iqbal Saripan M, Ramli AR. Computer-assisted diagnosis system for breast cancer in computed tomography laser mammography (CTLM). J Digit Imaging. 2017;30(6):796–811.
21. Doi K. Computer-aided diagnosis in medical imaging: historical review, current status and future potential. Comput Med Imaging Graph. 2007;31(4–5):198–211.
22. Bray F, Ren JS, Masuyer E, Ferlay J. Global estimates of cancer prevalence for 27 sites in the adult population in 2008. Int J Cancer. 2013;132(5):1133–45.
23. Dromain C, Thibault F, Muller S, Rimareix F, Delaloge S, Tardivon A, et al. Dual-energy contrast-enhanced digital mammography: initial clinical results. Eur Radiol. 2011;21(3):565–74.
24. Elpidio FG, Brasil LM, Lamas JM. Aid system to evaluation of breast calcification by case-based reasoning according to BI-RADS category. In: Mammography techniques and review. IntechOpen; 2015.
25. Izumori A, Takebe K, Sato A. Ultrasound findings and histological features of ductal carcinoma in situ detected by ultrasound examination alone. Breast Cancer. 2010;17(2):136–41.
26. Le Gal M, Ollivier L, Asselain B, Meunier M, Laurent M, Vielh P, et al. Mammographic features of 455 invasive lobular carcinomas. Radiology. 1992;185(3):705–8.
27. Gunhan-Bilgen I, Ustun EE, Memis A. Inflammatory breast carcinoma: mammographic, ultrasonographic, clinical, and pathologic findings in 142 cases. Radiology. 2002;223(3):829–38.
28. Grimm LJ, Rahbar H, Abdelmalak M, Hall AH, Ryser MD. Ductal carcinoma in situ: state-of-the-art review. Radiology. 2022;302(2):246–55.
29. Shin HJ, Kim HH, Huh MO, Kim MJ, Yi A, Kim H, et al. Correlation between mammographic and sonographic findings and prognostic factors in patients with node-negative invasive breast cancer. Br J Radiol. 2011;84(997):19–30.
30. Malherbe K, Bresser P. Association between ultrasound morphologic features and histopathological findings of lobular carcinoma. J Med Radiat Sci. 2019;66(3):177–83.
31. D'Orsi C. ACR BIRADS atlas. 5th ed. Springer, American College of Radiology; 2013.

32. Evans N, Lyons K. The use of ultrasound in the diagnosis of invasive lobular carcinoma of the breast less than 10 mm in size. Clin Radiol. 2000;55(4):261–3.
33. Mahoney MC, Newell MS. Screening MR imaging versus screening ultrasound: pros and cons. Magn Reson Imaging Clin N Am. 2013;21(3):495–508.
34. Dossus L, Benusiglio PR. Lobular breast cancer: incidence and genetic and non-genetic risk factors. Breast Cancer Res. 2015;17:37.
35. Lane DS, Smith RA. Cancer screening: patient and population strategies. Med Clin North Am. 2023;107(6):989–99.
36. Mukhtar TK, Yeates DR, Goldacre MJ. Breast cancer mortality trends in England and the assessment of the effectiveness of mammography screening: population-based study. J R Soc Med. 2013;106(6):234–42.
37. Marmot MG, Altman DG, Cameron DA, Dewar JA, Thompson SG, Wilcox M. The benefits and harms of breast cancer screening: an independent review. Br J Cancer. 2013;108(11):2205–40.
38. Kim JY, Jung EJ, Park T, Jeong SH, Jeong CY, Ju YT, et al. Prognostic importance of ultrasound BI-RADS classification in breast cancer patients. Jpn J Clin Oncol. 2015;45(5):411–5.
39. Berg WA, Gilbreath PL. Multicentric and multifocal cancer: whole-breast US in preoperative evaluation. Radiology. 2000;214(1):59–66.
40. Berg WA, Campassi C, Langenberg P, Sexton MJ. Breast imaging reporting and data system: inter- and intraobserver variability in feature analysis and final assessment. AJR Am J Roentgenol. 2000;174(6):1769–77.
41. Pestalozzi BC, Zahrieh D, Mallon E, Gusterson BA, Price KN, Gelber RD, et al. Distinct clinical and prognostic features of infiltrating lobular carcinoma of the breast: combined results of 15 international breast cancer study group clinical trials. J Clin Oncol. 2008;26(18):3006–14.
42. Shan J, Alam SK, Garra B, Zhang Y, Ahmed T. Computer-aided diagnosis for breast ultrasound using computerized BI-RADS features and machine learning methods. Ultrasound Med Biol. 2016;42(4):980–8.
43. Babu B, Dev B, Mohanapriya T, Shalini CNS. Bilateral mammary Paget disease in a young adult female. Radiol Case Rep. 2018;13(3):586–91.
44. Selinko VL, Middleton LP, Dempsey PJ. Role of sonography in diagnosing and staging invasive lobular carcinoma. J Clin Ultrasound. 2004;32(7):323–32.
45. Yi A, Kim HH, Shin HJ, Huh MO, Ahn SD, Seo BK. Radiation-induced complications after breast cancer radiation therapy: a pictorial review of multimodality imaging findings. Korean J Radiol. 2009;10(5):496–507.
46. Oucharqui S, Adil H, Benaissa E, Bssaibis F, En-Nafaa I, Maleb A, et al. Breast tuberculosis: a forgotten diagnosis. IDCases. 2021;26:e01341.
47. Stavros AT, Thickman D, Rapp CL, Dennis MA, Parker SH, Sisney GA. Solid breast nodules: use of sonography to distinguish between benign and malignant lesions. Radiology. 1995;196(1):123–34.
48. Fornage BD. Local and regional staging of invasive breast cancer with sonography: 25 years of practice at MD Anderson Cancer Center. Oncologist. 2014;19(1):5–15.
49. Dolan RT, Butler JS, Kell MR, Gorey TF, Stokes MA. Nipple discharge and the efficacy of duct cytology in evaluating breast cancer risk. Surgeon. 2010;8(5):252–8.
50. Soysal SD, Tzankov A, Muenst SE. Role of the tumor microenvironment in breast cancer. Pathobiology. 2015;82(3–4):142–52.
51. Moura C, Leite MI, Parreira R, Medeiros A. Primary breast lymphoma. J Surg Case Rep. 2020;2020(1):rjz405.
52. The radiology assistant: pathology of the male breast
53. Burnside ES, Sickles EA, Bassett LW, Rubin DL, Lee CH, Ikeda DM, et al. The ACR BI-RADS experience: learning from history. J Am Coll Radiol. 2009;6(12):851–60.
54. Alikhassi A, Akbari H, Yazdi SNM, Kia SA, Roozafzai F. Is breast background parenchymal enhancement on MRI related to BI-RADS score and follow-up rate? Adv Breast Cancer Res. 2018;07(01):15–22.
55. Mendelson EB, Harris KM, Doshi N, Tobon H. Infiltrating lobular carcinoma: mammographic patterns with pathologic correlation. AJR Am J Roentgenol. 1989;153(2):265–71.

56. Davoudi Y, Borhani B, Rad MP, Matin N. The role of Doppler sonography in distinguishing malignant from benign breast lesions. J Med Ultrasound. 2014;22(2):92–5.
57. Tang L, Jennings TA, Eaton JW. Mast cells mediate acute inflammatory responses to implanted biomaterials. Proc Natl Acad Sci USA. 1998;95(15):8841–6.
58. Watermann DO, Tempfer C, Hefler LA, Parat C, Stickeler E. Ultrasound morphology of invasive lobular breast cancer is different compared with other types of breast cancer. Ultrasound Med Biol. 2005;31(2):167–74.
59. Lee J. Practical and illustrated summary of updated BI-RADS for ultrasonography. Ultrasonography. 2017;36(1):71–81.
60. Tran TT, Hlaing M, Krause M. Point-of-care ultrasound: applications in low- and middle-income countries. Curr Anesthesiol Rep. 2021;11:1–7.
61. Gruszauskas NP, Drukker K, Giger ML, Sennett CA, Pesce LL. Performance of breast ultrasound computer-aided diagnosis: dependence on image selection. Acad Radiol. 2008;15(10):1234–45.
62. Schwab F, Redling K, Siebert M, Schotzau A, Schoenenberger CA, Zanetti-Dallenbach R. Inter- and intra-observer agreement in ultrasound BI-RADS classification and real-time Elastography Tsukuba score assessment of breast lesions. Ultrasound Med Biol. 2016;42(11):2622–9.
63. Dromain C, Balleyguier C, Adler G, Garbay JR, Delaloge S. Contrast-enhanced digital mammography. Eur J Radiol. 2009;69(1):34–42.
64. Park JM, Franken EA Jr, Garg M, Fajardo LL, Niklason LT. Breast tomosynthesis: present considerations and future applications. Radiographics. 2007;27(Suppl 1):S231–40.
65. Diebold T, Jacobi V, Scholz B, Hensel C, Solbach C, Kaufmann M, et al. Value of electrical impedance scanning (EIS) in the evaluation of BI-RADS III/IV/V-lesions. Technol Cancer Res Treat. 2005;4(1):93–7.
66. Muralidhar GS, Haygood TM, Stephens TW, Whitman GJ, Bovik AC, Markey MK. Computer-aided detection of breast cancer – have all bases been covered? Breast Cancer (Auckl). 2008;2:5–9.
67. Castellino RA. Computer aided detection (CAD): an overview. Cancer Imaging. 2005;5:17–9.
68. Acs B, Rantalainen M, Hartman J. Artificial intelligence as the next step towards precision pathology. J Intern Med. 2020;288(1):62–81.
69. Reiser I. Physics of stereo vs. tomosynthesis- guided breast biopsy; 2020

Benign Diseases of the Breast

2

Contents

K. Malherbe, *A Mammographers Guide: Radiological and Histopathological Guidelines*, https://doi.org/10.1007/978-3-031-84667-0_2

The term "benign" refers to noninvasive, self-limiting breast pathology, typically connected with normal hormonal fluctuations or other physiological changes within the breast. This differs from "malignancy," which refers to aberrant proliferation and expansion of the breast lobules and ducts. Benign breast disease can frequently be recognized using certain imaging criteria that indicate they do not require immediate treatment. Common imaging descriptors for benign conditions include phrases such as oval, well-rounded, well-encapsulated, large, bilateral, and unchanged from prior imaging [1–4].

2.1 Fibrocystic Breast Disease

Millions of women worldwide are diagnosed with fibrocystic breast disease, the most prevalent benign form of breast disease. The way this disease is evaluated, treated, and functions is largely dependent on certain hormonal aspects. A variety of benign breast abnormalities, including tumors, trauma, mastalgia, and nipple discharge, are collectively referred to as benign breast disease. The benign lesions indicated above are not linked to an elevated risk of malignancy; but, in particular in histological and clinical situations, they are linked to a 50% chance of developing breast cancer. Upon clinical evaluation and imaging, both benign and malignant breast diseases are associated with a palpable tumor. Clinical findings include symptoms like thickening, discomfort, nipple discharge, and skin dimpling (peau d'orange) [5].

Mammograms and ultrasound are the most often used investigative techniques to assess for these clinical abnormalities.

Hormonal imbalances can cause fibrocystic alterations in the primary components of the breast. The breast's stroma, ducts, and lobules are some of these parts. Estradiol and progesterone plasma levels have cyclical surges that are directly correlated with glandular breast tissue during the reproductive age.

Benign cysts are typically mobile within the glandular breast tissue, chest wall, and skin and are rubber-like in texture. Except for inflammatory type cysts, discomfort and tenderness experienced by a patient are either absent or mild. Most patients present with multiple cysts upon further clinical and diagnostic evaluation [6].

Various subtypes of cysts are known, including hyperplastic fibrous cysts, adenosis, and papillomatosis (see Fig. 2.1). These types of cysts are usually found in the upper outer quadrants of the breast, as well as in the central margins. The texture upon evaluation ranges from a firm texture to multiple subcentimeter cysts.

Fibroadenomas present in varied sizes with a common oval-shaped, well-defined margin. As with cysts, fibroadenomas are mobile upon evaluation and are often multiple, occurring either simultaneously or over a specified period.

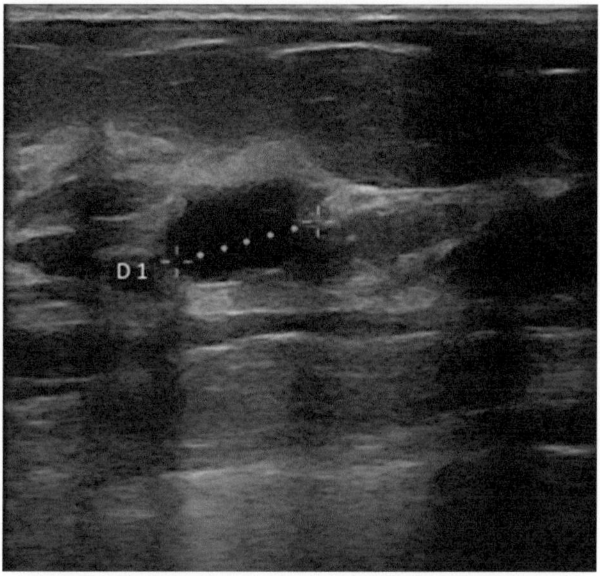

Fig. 2.1 Ultrasound evaluation of a cyst within the breast using B-mode imaging. Benign cysts appear oval-shaped, well-circumscribed, with a thin echogenic capsule surrounding it. The overlying tissue is also displaced away from the fluid collection, which is also an indication of benignancy

Nipple discharge is associated with ductal ectasia, intraductal papilloma, or in rare instances, carcinoma [4, 7, 8].

2.1.1 Pathophysiology and Histopathology

Mammary gland development, maturation, and differentiation act upon the hormonal and growth factor changes affecting the stromal and epithelial cells.

During the late proliferative phase, glandular tissue evolves to hyperplastic stages such as sclerosing adenosis or lobular hyperplasia. This state of hyperplasia, if associated with a 2% prevalence of Ki67 cells, has a twofold increased incidence for the development of breast cancer. Various types of benign breast diseases exist, such as hyperplasia, cysts, fibroadenomas, sclerosing adenosis, and mastitis.

There is a limited pathological consensus regarding the histopathological appearance of benign breast disease. The main features are an extracellular matrix of collagen, pericanalicular patterns of stromal cells with the presence of florid epithelial hyperplasia.

During the menopausal phase, fibroadenomas involute, which affects dense collagen stroma and atrophic glands. Cystic changes derive from the terminal duct lobular unit (TDLU). Due to the expansion of the efferent ductules of the TDLU, cysts form as a result of fluid accumulation in these structures. The lining appears flat with a myoepithelial layer present [5].

2.1.2 Clinical Evaluation and Imaging

Nodularity in young women less than 30 years of age may have management with clinical surveillance and short-term follow-up examination in 2–3 months. An investigation may be necessary if the lump has changed on review or if, at the initial presentation, there is a new change in her breasts. Nodularity or thickening that is asymmetric in women over the age of 30 years, further investigation utilizing mammography and ultrasound, is warranted.

Short-term follow-up is an important part of the management of nodularity so that the progression in size of a mass of nodularity or other associated findings (e.g., skin or nipple changes) is detected.

Mammography with ultrasound examination is required for all discrete palpable lesions in women over 35 to distinguish cysts from solid lesions. Complex cysts containing both fluid and solid matter require biopsy. For solid lesions, radiographically or ultrasonically directed core biopsy provides further information regarding the presence or absence of malignancy [9, 10].

2.1.3 Treatment and Management

Due to the role of estrogen and progesterone treatments, promoting fibrocystic changes in the breast, metformin has been suggested as a treatment method to reduce the excessive cell proliferation caused by associated hormones. For patients presenting with mastalgia, the first-line options are lifestyle changes. Other suggestions are the use of a supportive bra, as well as altering the dose of hormone replacement therapy regimen. Analgesics such as aspirin and ibuprofen are options.

Researchers have proposed that a deficiency in prostaglandin E and its precursor gamma-linolenic acid (GLA) increase the sensitivity of breasts during the luteal phase of the menstrual cycle. GLA is subsequently also the active component of evening primrose oil.

Despite not having proven efficacy in previous studies, the use of evening primrose oil is warranted as supportive measures if pain persists despite treatment and advice. A 3- to 6-month period is the suggested timeframe to observe the desired effect.

If breast pain persists for more than 6 months and disrupts daily activities, other therapies such as tamoxifen, bromocriptine, or danazol can be options. Due to the recurrent nature and long duration of these symptoms, several months of treatment is necessary [4, 9, 11].

2.1.4 Clinical Advice for Patients

- Use over-the-counter pain relievers such as acetaminophen or ibuprofen.
- Apply warm or cool compresses to breasts when most painful.
- Wear a comfortable, supportive bra.
- Avoid large amounts of salt or fat in the diet, which some women find can worsen symptoms.
- Consider an oral contraceptive.
- Check thyroid levels and suggest the use of iodine.
- Consider vitamin E, evening primrose oil, and B vitamins.

2.2 Fibroadenoma

A fibroadenoma is a painless, unilateral, benign (noncancerous) breast tumor that is a solid, not fluid-filled, lump. It occurs most commonly in women between 14 and 35 but can be found at any age. Fibroadenomas shrink after menopause and, therefore, are less common in postmenopausal women. Fibroadenomas are often referred to as a "breast mouse" due to their high mobility. Fibroadenomas are a marble-like mass comprising both epithelial and stromal tissues located under the skin of the breast. These firm, rubbery masses with regular borders are often variable in size [9, 12–14].

2.2.1 Pathophysiology and Histopathology

Fibroadenoma arises from stromal and epithelial connective tissue cells that are functionally and mechanically important in the breast. These tissues contain receptors for both estrogen and progesterone. For this reason, fibroadenomas tend to proliferate during pregnancy because of excessive production of female reproductive hormones. Hormone sensitivity causes excessive proliferation of breast connective tissues. Mediator complex subunit 12 (*MED12*) gene is also important in the pathophysiology of fibroadenomas [9, 12–14].

A fibroadenoma is a well-circumscribed, nonencapsulated lesion with pushing borders that does not infiltrate the adjacent breast parenchyma. They are characterized by a cellular proliferation of stroma and glands (benign breast ducts). The ratio between stroma and glands is relatively constant throughout the entire lesion. The stroma is uniform, hypovascular, and composed of spindle-shaped cells with bland oval to elongated nuclei. There is no stromal cell pleomorphism present. Smooth muscle, cartilage, and bone may be identified in the stroma. Stromal mitosis, although rare, can be seen, especially in fibroadenomas of younger women, and does not indicate malignancy. In older women, the stroma can be hyalinized.

The glands in a fibroadenoma consist of the normal bi-cell layer in breast ducts. The inner glandular layer comprises cuboidal to columnar-shaped cells with uniform nuclei. The inner cell layer is supported by an outer myoepithelial cell layer. The myoepithelial layer is intact throughout the entire lesion, designating a fibroadenoma's benign nature. Benign alterations such as usual ductal hyperplasia, apocrine metaplasia, squamous metaplasia, cystic changes, and sclerosing adenosis can involve the epithelium. Calcifications can also be in the glands. In pregnancy, the epithelium may show lactation changes [9, 12–14].

2.2.2 Clinical Evaluation and Imaging

Age is the most important factor in the incidence of fibroadenoma. Therefore, when obtaining a medical history, age is the most important factor which should be considered. A family history of breast cancer is also significant. Female patients who have first-degree relatives with breast cancer should be monitored and observed more carefully for malignant features than patients without this family history. Fibroadenoma most commonly occurs in the upper outer quadrant of the breast. On physical examination, it has the following features:

- Non-tender or painless.
- Mobile.
- Solitary.
- Rapidly growing solid lump with rubbery consistency and regular borders.

Fibroadenoma on a mammogram appears as a distinct area from other breast tissue, with smooth, round edges (see Fig. 2.2). Mammographic features of fibroadenomas are variable from a well-circumscribed discrete oval mass hypodense or isodense of breast glandular tissue to a mass with macrolobulation or partially obscured margins. Involuting fibroadenomas in older, typically postmenopausal, patients may contain calcification, often producing the classic, coarse popcorn calcification appearance [9, 12–14].

Ultrasound uses sound waves to detect the features of fibroadenomas in women younger than 35 years of age. Ultrasound easily differentiates solid from the cystic

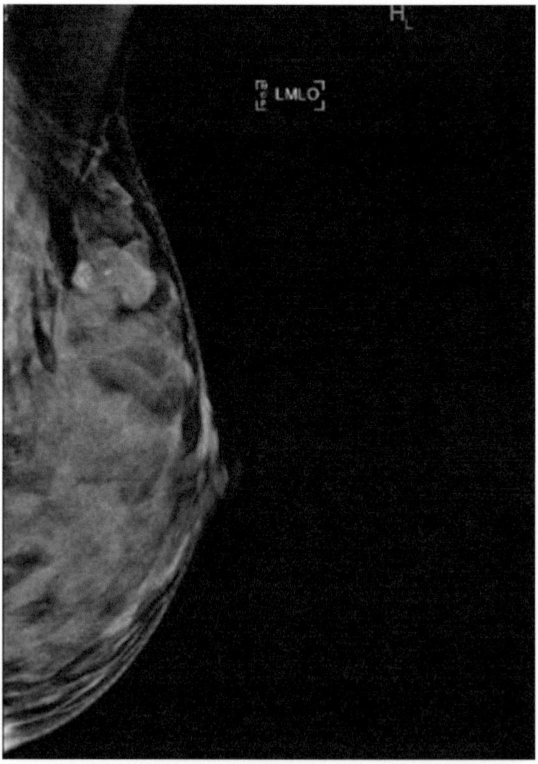

Fig. 2.2 MLO left mammogram of a fibroadenoma
The view indicates an oval-shaped, well-rounded mass in the upper outer quadrant, and further imaging with ultrasound would help determine the echogenicity and internal architecture of the visualized mass. Note the dense-type breast tissue (ACR Type D) which is typically associated with fibroadenomas

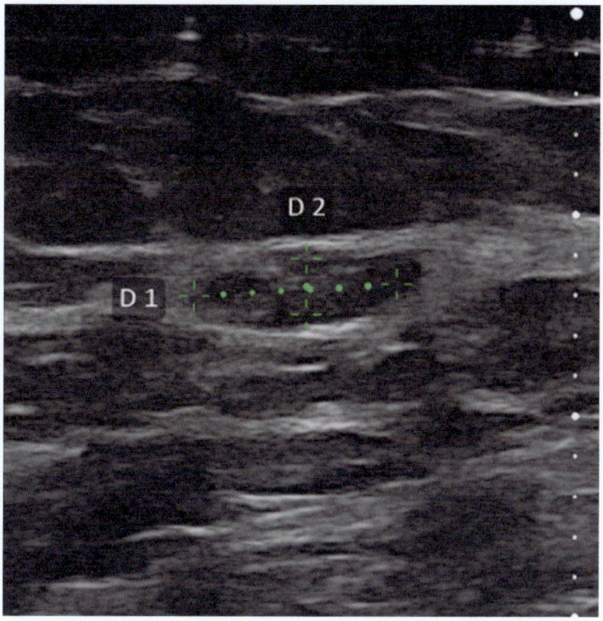

Fig. 2.3 Ultrasound appearance of a fibroadenoma
Using B-mode imaging, a fibroadenoma typically presents as an oval-shaped, well-circumscribed mass with a thin echogenic capsule. The mass also indicates no signs of surrounding invasion into adjacent breast tissue, and the internal echogenicity would appear homogenous and smooth, with no signs of necrosis or macrocalcifications present

masses. On ultrasound, a fibroadenoma is typically seen as a well-circumscribed, round to ovoid, or macrolobulated mass with generally uniform hypo echogenicity (see Fig. 2.3). If necessary, a minimally invasive biopsy may be performed via a core needle biopsy [9, 12–14].

2.2.3 Treatment and Management

Fibroadenomas usually do not require surgical intervention. They eventually fade away, but if they are really large and putting pressure on other breast tissues, they ought to be removed. Since the lesions are benign and carry no long-term risk of cancer, many girls choose not to have the operation. Breast form is also distorted by surgery.

If the fibroadenoma is large and keeps growing, doctors may choose to remove it. Surgical intervention is indicated when there is a patient's desire, rapid growth, or size larger than 2 cm. A fibroadenoma can be surgically removed in two ways:

1. Lumpectomy, also known as excisional biopsy: During this operation, the fibroadenoma is removed by the surgeon and sent to a lab for additional analysis.
2. Cryoablation: Surgeons use a cryoprobe to freeze and destroy the cellular structure of fibroadenoma. A core needle biopsy must be performed before cryoablation to confirm the fibroadenoma [9, 12–14]

2.3 Gynecomastia

Male breast development follows a similar pattern to female breast development. During puberty, a complicated hormonal interplay occurs, resulting in the growth and maturation of the adult female breast [9, 12–14].

In early fetal development, epithelial cells generated from the epidermis of the area planned to become the areola proliferate into ducts that connect to the nipple on the skin's surface. In late gestation, the blind ends of these ducts develop into alveolar structures. The infantile breast regresses until puberty as fetal prolactin, placental estrogen, and progesterone levels decrease [9, 12–14].

During the larche in females, the breast bud makes its initial clinical appearance, and the ducts expand and divide, giving rise to club-shaped terminal end buds that eventually form alveolar buds. The type 1 lobule is formed by the clustering of approximately a dozen alveolar buds around a terminal duct. The type 1 lobule will develop into types 2 and 3 lobules, known as ductules. In type 2 and 3 lobules, the number of alveolar buds can reach 50 and 80, respectively. The entire differentiation process takes years after puberty, and if pregnancy is not attained, it may never be finished. On the contrary, increased testosterone concentrations during puberty normally prevent additional breast development [9, 12–14].

2.3.1 Pathophysiology and Histopathology

2.3.1.1 Physiological Gynecomastia

Gynecomastia, or male breast development, can occur naturally during three stages of life. The first takes place immediately after birth in both males and females. This is partly due to high fetal blood levels of estradiol and progesterone (made by the mother), which stimulate breast tissue in the infant. Another process is the enhanced conversion of steroid hormone precursors to sex steroids, as well as increased androgen aromatization, caused by the new-born surge of luteinizing hormone (LH). Neonatal gynecomastia can last for several weeks after birth and is accompanied with a milky breast discharge known as "witch's milk" [2].

Puberty is the second period when gynecomastia can arise biologically. By the age of 14, up to 60% of males have gynecomastia that can be clinically detected. Although it is typically bilateral, it is frequently asymmetrical and can occur unilaterally [9, 12–16]. Pubertal gynecomastia often resolves within 3 years of start [2]. During early puberty, the pituitary gland secretes gonadotropins at night and increases testosterone production in the testicles in the early morning. However, serum estrogen concentrations stay above prepubertal levels throughout the day. Boys with pubertal gynecomastia have a lower androgen-to-estrogen ratio compared to those without it. Another study found higher aromatase activity in the skin fibroblasts of boys with gynecomastia, which is known as the process [13], which causes pubertal gynecomastia.

The third age range in which gynecomastia is frequently seen is during older age (>60 years) [9, 12–14].

2.3.1.2 Pathological Gynecomastia

Pathological gynecomastia is due to an increase in the circulating and/or local breast tissue ratio of estrogen to androgen.

Breast development in adult males requires estrogen, while androgens have antiproliferative effects. An imbalance exists between estrogen and androgens, preventing growth of breast tissue. Increased estrogen levels increase glandular proliferation through direct stimulation and suppression of LH, decreasing testosterone secretion by the testes and exaggerating the high estrogen-to-androgen ratio. The same hormones affecting female breast tissue can cause gynecomastia in males [15].

Testicular tumors can increase blood estrogen levels through estrogen overproduction, androgen overproduction, and secretion of hCG stimulating normal Leydig cells. These tumors, including Leydig cell tumors, constitute 1–3% of all testicular tumors and typically occur in men aged 20–60. In adults, elevated estrogen levels, palpable testicular mass, and gynecomastia suggest a testicular tumor. Leydig cell tumors can be benign or malignant and may metastasize to other lymph nodes. Other tumors include Sertoli Cell tumors, Granulose cell tumors, adrenal tumors, gonadal germ cell tumor, and hepatocellular carcinoma [15].

Men with end-stage renal disease may have reduced testosterone and elevated gonadotropins, leading to increased breast development. Gynecomastia in liver disease, particularly cirrhosis, is associated with increased SHBG binding to testosterone more than estrogen. The etiology of gynecomastia is unclear, but current data is conflicting. Thyrotoxicosis is associated with gynecomastia, as it stimulates estrogen production and increases LH, which stimulates testosterone aromatization. This leads to an elevated free estrogen to testosterone ratio.

Gynecomastia is linked to spinal cord disorders, low testosterone levels, and testicular atrophy, leading to hypogonadism and infertility. Refeeding gynecomastia involves breast development in men recovering from malnutrition, but the exact cause remains elusive. HIV patients also develop gynecomastia due to androgen deficiency [15].

About 20% of gynecomastia is caused by medications or exogenous chemicals, which can increase estrogen effects through intrinsic estrogen-like properties, increased endogenous estrogen production, or an excess of an estrogen precursor. Examples include contact with estrogen vaginal creams, estrogen-containing embalming creams, topical estrogen sprays, recreational use of marijuana, heroin, methadone, amphetamines, and herbals with estrogen-like structures. Digitalis, which binds to estrogen receptors, may also cause gynecomastia. The appearance of gynecomastia is often observed in body builders and athletes.

Gynecomastia patients should have serum testosterone, estradiol, LH, and hCG measured. Further testing should be tailored based on the patient's history, physical examination, and initial tests. Elevated beta hCG or hCG suggests neoplasm, and a testicular ultrasound is warranted. Low testosterone and LH indicate primary hypogonadism, with Klinefelter syndrome requiring a karyotype for definitive diagnosis. Elevated testosterone and LH suggest androgen resistance, and liver, kidney, and thyroid function should be assessed. If breast tissue suggests malignancy, a biopsy is performed, especially in patients with Klinefelter syndrome [15].

2.3.2 Clinical Evaluation and Imaging

When performing breast imaging on males, always follow the rule: "If it is not normal, gynecomastia, or classically benign, it needs a biopsy."

Fig. 2.5 is an example of normal male mammogram image. The MLO image on the left shows normal skin, a nipple, and some connective tissue behind it (see Fig. 2.5).

The right B-mode ultrasound image also demonstrates the normal sonographic appearance of male fibroglandular breast tissue in the retroareolar space [9, 12–14].

There are three image patterns related to the male breast:

- Nodular glandular (acute florid phase) (see Fig. 2.4).
- Dendritic (chronic fibrotic phase).
- Diffuse glandular.

It may be more visible in the top outside quadrant, but more significantly, it blends into the surrounding fat.

If you see the mammogram on the left as a woman's breast rather than a man's, you might remark that there is an ill-defined mass and conclude that this is a malignancy.

However, in a man this indistinct border is a sign of a gynecomastia [9, 12–14].

2.3.3 Treatment and Management

If the gynecomastia is severe, does not resolve, has a recent onset (less than 6 months), and does not have a curable underlying cause, several medical therapy may be tried. There are three types of medicinal treatment for gynecomastia: androgens (testosterone, dihydrotestosterone, danazol), anti-estrogens (clomiphene citrate, tamoxifen), and aromatase inhibitors like letrozole and anastrozole.

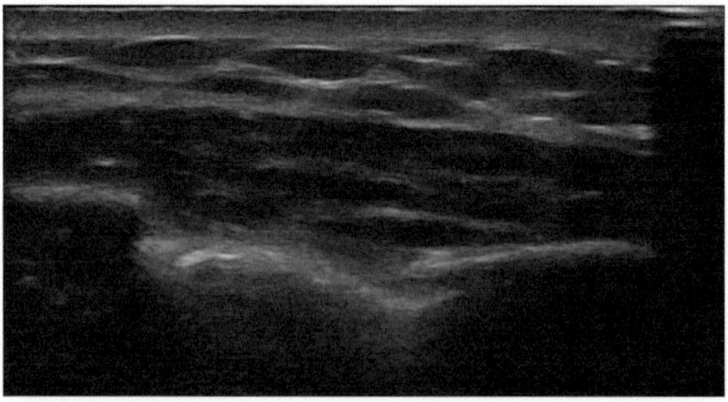

Fig. 2.4 Left B-mode ultrasound image of a male breast
Small areas of fibro glandular tissue present (nodular), and the patient was presenting with breast tenderness
Note the appearance of the pectoralis muscle deep to the subcutaneous soft tissue, seen in male patients

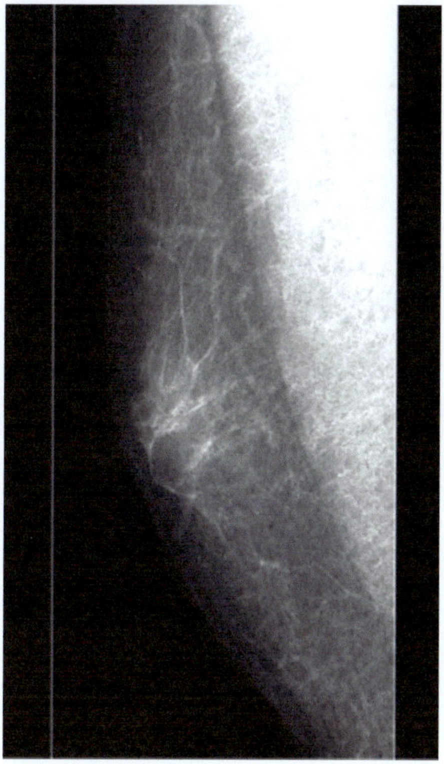

Fig. 2.5 Right MLO image of gynecomastia This demonstrates a male breast with a nodular glandular pattern of gynecomastia with a fan-shaped density emerging from the nipple

Once gynecomastia is established, testosterone treatment for hypogonadal men with gynecomastia frequently fails to result in breast retraction. Testosterone treatment may theoretically cause gynecomastia by aromatizing to estradiol; however, this side effect is rare and temporary. However, there is limited evidence to support its use to particularly treat gynecomastia in hypogonadism [9, 12–14].

When medical therapy fails, particularly in situations of long-standing gynecomastia, when the gynecomastia interferes with the patient's everyday activities, or when there is a suspicion of breast cancer, surgical therapy is recommended. On the other hand, surgical therapy for pubertal gynecomastia should be delayed until after puberty to reduce the risk of recurring gynecomastia. Surgery should also be avoided until the underlying cause of gynecomastia has been addressed or cured. Surgical treatment includes glandular tissue removal and, if necessary, liposuction, ideally using a customized method. Nowadays, minimally invasive surgery is possible, which may be associated with fewer problems and a faster recovery. If cancer is suspected, a histological study is required.When medical therapy fails, particularly in situations of long-standing gynecomastia, when the gynecomastia interferes with the patient's everyday activities, or when there is a suspicion of breast cancer, surgical therapy is recommended. On the other hand, surgical therapy for pubertal gynecomastia should be delayed until after puberty to reduce the risk of recurring gynecomastia. Surgery should also be avoided until the underlying cause of gynecomastia has been addressed or cured. Surgical treatment includes glandular tissue removal and, if necessary, liposuction, ideally using a customized method. Nowadays, minimally invasive surgery is possible, which may be associated with fewer problems and a faster recovery. If cancer is suspected, a histological study is required [9, 12–14, 17, 18].

2.4 Phyllodes Tumor of Benign Type

Phyllodes tumor is a rare fibroepithelial neoplasm accounting for less than 1% of all breast tumors. It has a leaf-like architecture and infiltrating margins with marked stromal overgrowth and hypercellularity. The behavior of phyllodes tumors ranges from benign and locally recurrent to malignant and metastatic. The accepted histological classification is into benign, borderline, and malignant subtypes, according to features such as tumor margins (pushing or infiltrative), stromal overgrowth, tumor necrosis, cellular atypia, and the number of mitoses per high power field. However, histological grading has been shown to correlate poorly with tumor behavior, though the multiplicity of differing grading systems makes it difficult to be certain whether this effect is in part a result of disparities in approach [9, 12–14, 17, 18]:

- Incidence rate of 2.1 per 1 million women.
- Constitutes 1% of breast tumors.
- Benign phyllodes tumor most common (60–75%), followed by borderline (15–26%) and malignant (8–20%) tumors.
- Average age 40–50 years.
- Benign phyllodes tumor occurs at a younger age compared with borderline and malignant phyllodes tumors.
- Can occur rarely in pediatric age group and male.

2.4.1 Pathophysiology and Histopathology

- Biphasic lesion with epithelial stromal interaction involved in tumorigenesis.
- Loss of epithelial interaction in the stromal component is believed to lead to malignant progression (see Fig. 2.8).
- Areas resembling well-differentiated liposarcoma in phyllodes tumor lack CDK4 and MDM2 expression / gene amplification as seen in primary well-differentiated liposarcoma [9, 12–14, 17, 18].

2.4.2 Clinical Evaluation and Imaging

Phyllodes tumors typically appear as a clinically insignificant mass that may be expanding quickly. A long-standing breast lesion may suddenly get larger, triggering presentation. Although improved breast awareness and the influence of screening have led to a tendency toward presentation at reduced tumor sizes, the size at presentation is generally bigger than for fibroadenoma. Bluish discoloration, dilated veins, and pressure necrosis can appear on the skin layer above. Asian and Caucasian people in Latin America have greater prevalence rates. Most cases occur in women between the ages of 35 and 55 (around 20 years after fibroadenoma). There is no clinically discernible difference between phyllodes tumor and fibroadenoma or other benign breast lesions, although some clinical symptoms may increase the suspicion. The phyllodes diagnosis should be considered upon evaluation of larger fibroadenomas [9, 12–14, 17, 18].

Mammography and ultrasonography are the mainstays of routine imaging of breast lumps. Phyllodes tumor often mimics fibroadenoma at mammography (see Figs. 2.5, 2.6, 2.7, 2.8, 2.9, and 2.10), commonly appearing as a large, well-circumscribed, oval or lobulated mass with rounded borders, which may show a lucent halo or coarse microcalcifications. Ultrasonography typically shows an inhomogeneous, solid appearing mass with low-level internal echoes, smooth walls, and good through transmission (see Figs. 2.6, 2.7, and 2.11). Identification of a cyst within a solid lesion by ultrasound is highly suggestive of phyllodes tumor [9, 12–14, 17, 18].

The role of MRI has not been fully elucidated, but dynamic enhancement patterns may be helpful for the diagnosis of larger tumors (>3 cm). Other experimental

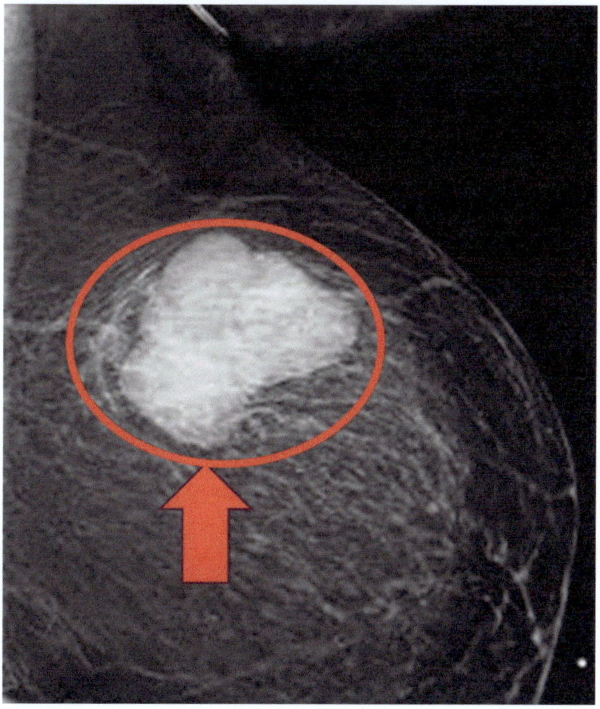

Fig. 2.6 Left mammogram image of a phyllodes tumor CC image indicating a solid multilobular hyperdense mass in the superiolateral aspect of the breast

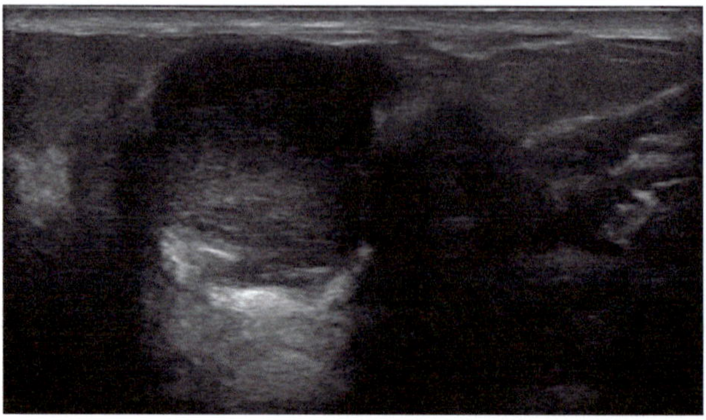

Fig. 2.7 Ultrasound of a 14-year-old female indicates an oval-shaped well-circumscribed mass with posterior acoustic enhancement. Internal echogenicity indicates a smooth homogenous texture

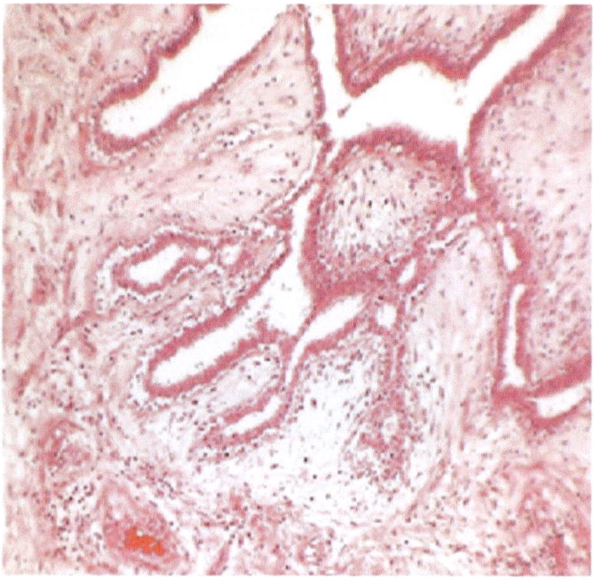

Fig. 2.8 Histological image of a phyllodes tumor
Above image indicates hypercellular stroma with epithelial elements. Stromal spindle cells show no signs of pleomorphism or mitotic activity [19]

approaches include proton magnetic resonance spectroscopy and scintimammography. At present, however, many phyllodes tumors cannot be distinguished from fibroadenomas on radiological grounds, nor can benign and malignant variants be reliably differentiated, although one study found tumors larger than 3 cm in diameter are more likely to be malignant [9, 12–14, 17, 18].

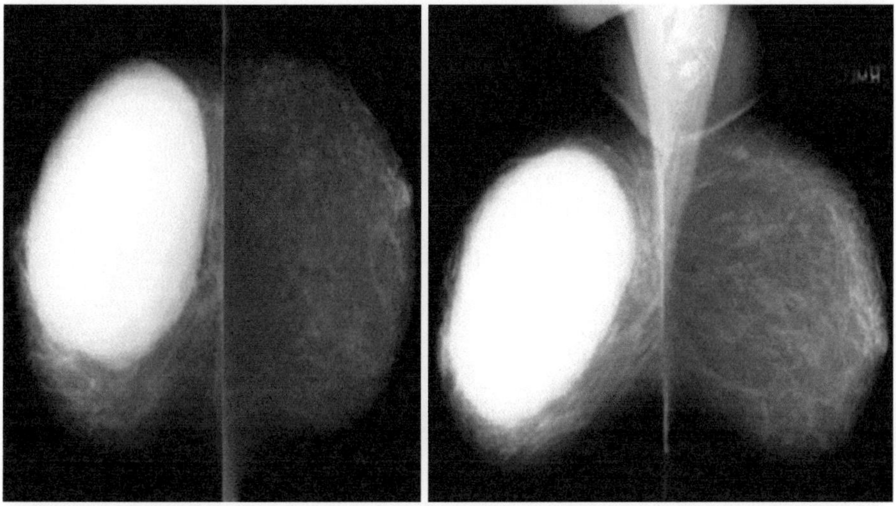

Fig. 2.9 Right CC view demonstrating a phyllodes tumor
Above figure indicates a large multilobular mass with solid contents in the central aspect of the breast [19]

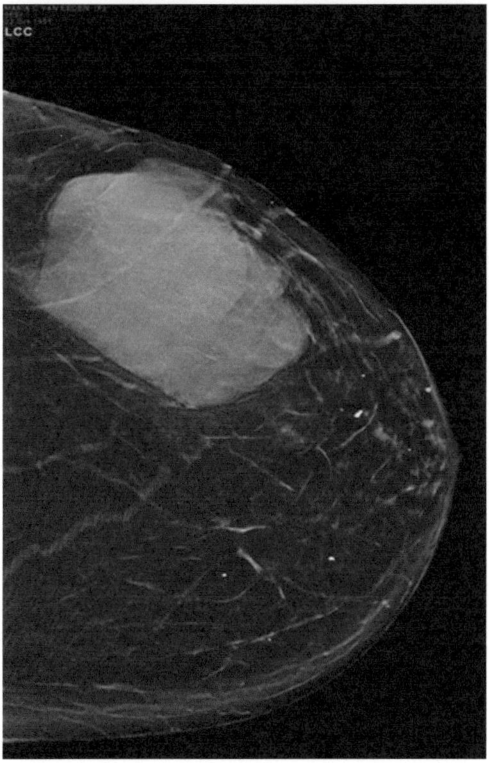

Fig. 2.10 Left CC view of a phyllodes tumor

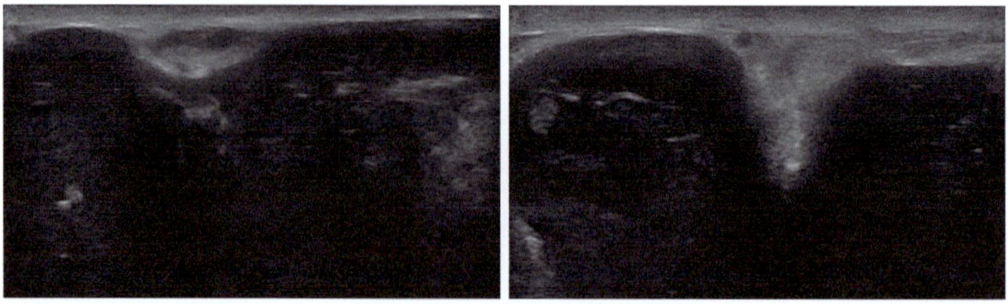

Fig. 2.11 B-mode ultrasound image of large phyllodes tumor
Image with Color Doppler box indicates a complex, multilobular mass with mixed internal echogenicity. Signs of internal cystic necrosis are noted and small areas of microcalcifications

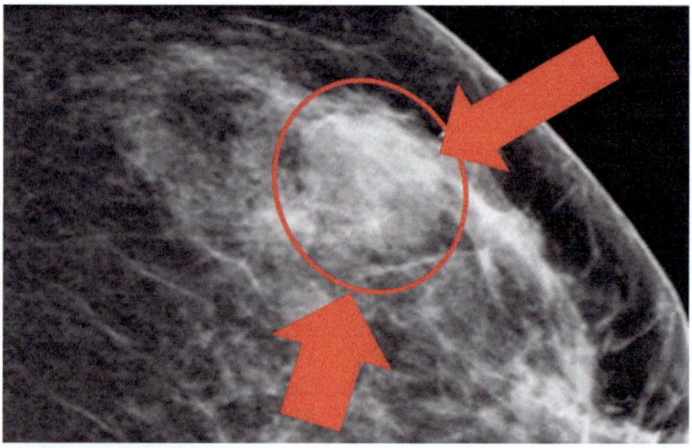

Fig. 2.12 Mammogram image of an oval-shaped mass
Left magnified CC mammogram view indicates an isodense oval-shaped region

2.4.3 Treatment and Management

Treatment can be either wide local excision or mastectomy to achieve histologically clear margins. After the treatment of phyllodes tumor, long-term follow-up by the primary care providers/nurse practitioner is necessary to detect local and distant relapse [9, 12–14, 17, 18].

2.5 Hyperplasia of Benign Type

Hyperplasia occurs when there is an increase in the number of cells lining the ducts (tubes that carry milk to the nipple) or lobules (milk-producing glands) of the breast.

When hyperplasia occurs in the ducts, it is referred to as ductal hyperplasia. Ductal hyperplasia can be either “usual” or “atypical” (see Fig. 2.12). Atypical typically refers to a precursor for malignancy in patients. When hyperplasia occurs in the lobules, it is referred to atypical lobular hyperplasia. Usual ductal hyperplasia, also known as epithelial hyperplasia, is a benign proliferation of normal cells in breast ducts and lobules. The mean age of patients with epithelial hyperplasia is 54 years [9, 12–14, 17, 18].

2.5.1 Pathophysiology and Histopathology

- Breast ducts and lobules usually lined by a single outer layer of myoepithelial cells and a single inner layer of epithelial/luminal cells.
- In usual ductal hyperplasia, there are an increased number of myoepithelial and luminal cell types that fill and distend ducts and lobules 2.
- No epithelial cell atypia [9, 12–14, 17, 18].

2.6 Changes Before or During Surgery and Treatment

2.6.1 During Radiation Therapy

The below table indicates the early, intermediate, and late signs of radiation therapy [20, 21] (Table 2.1).

2.6.1.1 Breast Edema

During the acute period after irradiation, inflammatory markers are induced, and the expression of these proteins contributes to increased vascular permeability of breast tissue. Breast edema that manifests as skin and trabecular thickening appears generally in the first several weeks after completion of radiation therapy. Initially, there is engorgement of the dermal as well as of the intramammary lymphatics (trabecular thickening). This edema usually resolves over a period of weeks, months, or sometimes years. Radiographically, an irradiated breast with skin and trabecular thickening appears denser as compared to the contralateral normal breast (see Fig. 2.13) [20, 21].

2.6.1.2 Fat Necrosis

Breast fat necrosis exhibits various profiles according to the process of nonpurulent inflammation and absorption (see Fig. 2.14). Intimal arterial damage caused by

Table 2.1 Complications post-radiation therapy

Post-radiation	Time	Complications
Early	Weeks to months	Skin thickening with breast edema Fat necrosis Dystrophic calcifications Radiation-induced pneumonia Pleural effusion
Intermediate	Months to years	Skin retraction with breast fibrosis Glandular atrophy Lactation difficulty Overlying bone fracture Pulmonary fibrosis Pericardial disease
Late	More than 10 years	Cardiomyopathy Radiation-induced malignancy

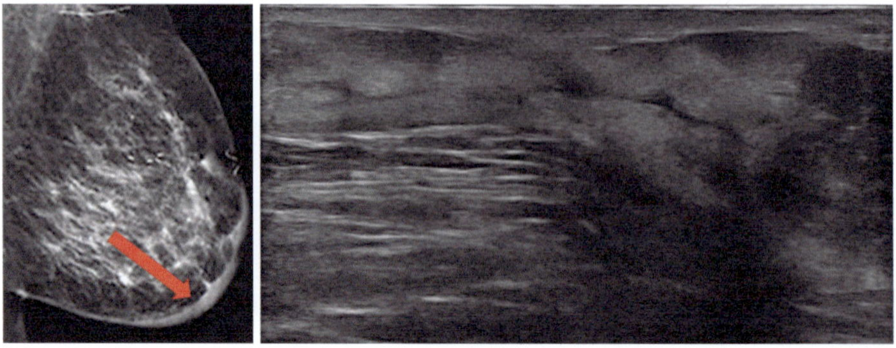

Fig. 2.13 Mammogram and ultrasound image during radiation therapy
Bilateral mammogram image shows markedly thickened skin and retraction from the left breast during radiation therapy. Internal surgical staples are also noted within the breast tissue. B-mode ultrasound indicates localized swelling and edema of the subcutaneous soft tissue

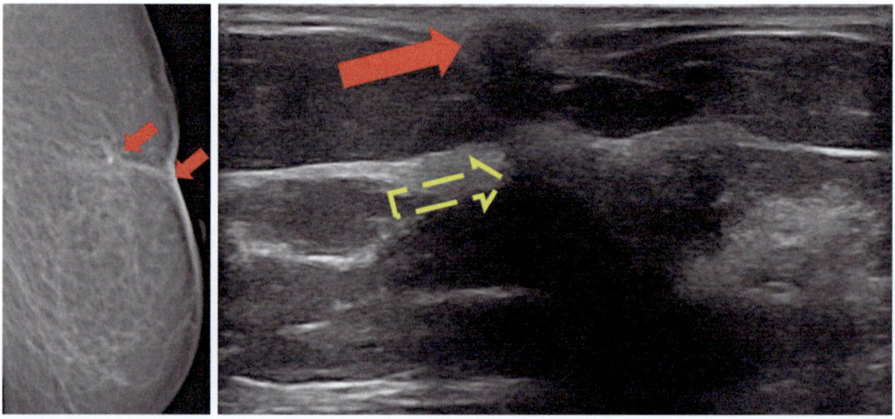

Fig. 2.14 Scar tissue appearance on mammogram and ultrasound
Left MLO mammogram image shows architectural distortion and retraction of the breast tissue alongside surgical staples. Malignancy has a similar appearance, and thus histology is required to confirm scar tissue is present
Corresponding B-mode ultrasound image indicates a localized area of tissue necrosis (dotted arrow) which coincides with the area of previous surgical incision site marked on the skin surface (arrow)

radiation exposure combined with surgical damage may result in tissue necrosis directly or indirectly.

Mammographically, the presence of a radiolucent oil cyst, round opacity, asymmetrical opacity, heterogeneity of the subcutaneous tissue, dystrophic calcification, clustered pleomorphic microcalcification, or the presence of a spiculated mass is noted. An ultrasound (US) examination can demonstrate the presence of a solid or anechoic mass with posterior acoustic shadowing or enhancement and can demonstrate the presence of a cyst with a mural nodule or internal echo or increased echogenicity of the subcutaneous tissue [20, 21].

2.6.1.3 Radiation-Induced Calcifications

Radiation-induced calcifications are benign dystrophic calcifications that are due to a combination of surgical trauma and radiation exposure. The calcifications are generally large and irregular in pattern, with central lucency and calcifications that always occur at the site of surgery (see Fig. 2.15). In addition, it is common for sutures to calcify after radiation therapy. Calcified sutures are usually characteristic as the calcified sutures are equally spaced along the suture line and the presence of calcified knots is frequently evident [20, 21].

2.6.1.4 Long-Term Effects Include Glandular Atrophy

Figure 2.16 refers to significant loss of overall breast volume along with atrophy of the fibroglandular tissue when compared to the contralateral right side.

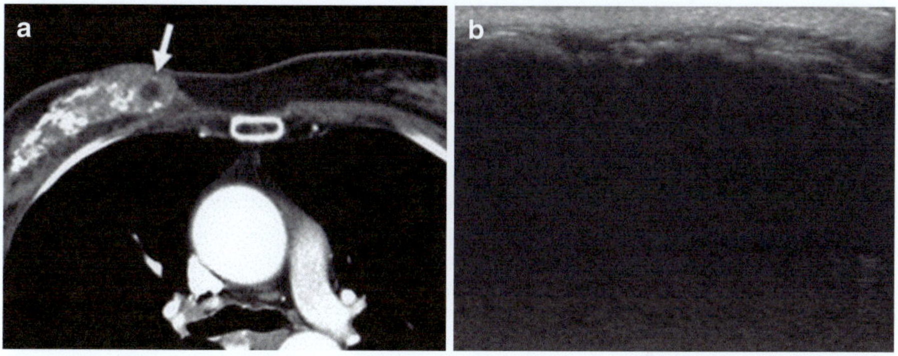

Fig. 2.15 Axial CT during radiation therapy
Axial CT of the chest wall (bone window) indicates large coarse calcifications within the overlying soft tissue of the breast. Corresponding B-mode ultrasound shows dense calcifications with strong posterior acoustic shadowing and hyperechoic rim, typical of coarse-type calcifications [20, 21]

Fig. 2.16 Mammogram demonstrating long-term effects of radiation therapy Bilateral MLO image indicates dense-type breast tissue and asymmetry of the left breast and reduction in size and glandular contents in comparison to the contralateral right side [20, 21]

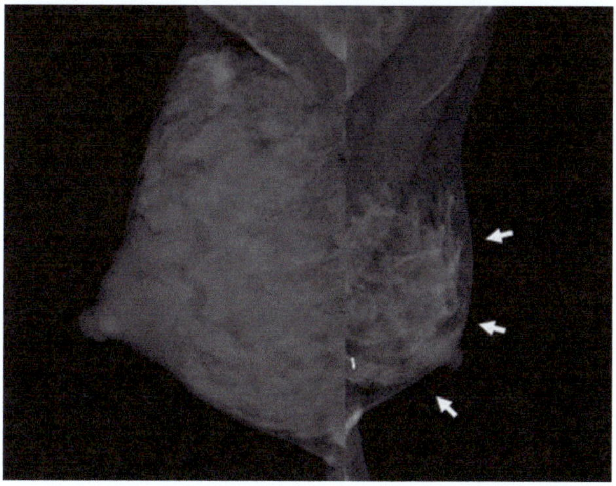

2.6.1.5 Radiation-Induced Malignancy

During concurrent sessions of radiation therapy, there is the possibility of reoccurrence of malignancy, as seen in Fig. 2.17.

2.6.1.6 Common Pitfall

Radiation-induced breast edema shows similar imaging findings as the serious condition of inflammatory breast cancer, with a diffusely enlarged breast with trabecular and skin thickening as depicted on mammography and US. However, inflammatory breast cancer shows the presence of a malignant mass lesion within the edematous breast parenchyma, and inflammatory breast cancer may be accompanied with a coexisting metastatic lymph node in the ipsilateral axillary area (see Fig. 2.18). In contrast, radiation-induced breast edema does not show a coexisting malignant mass and metastatic axillary lymph node; radiation-induced breast edema slowly resolves and may progress to benign breast fibrosis [20, 21].

2.6.2 Following a Mastectomy/Lumpectomy

As seen in Fig. 2.19, following surgery of the left breast, there is local organization at the site of surgical excision, with visible coarse calcifications.

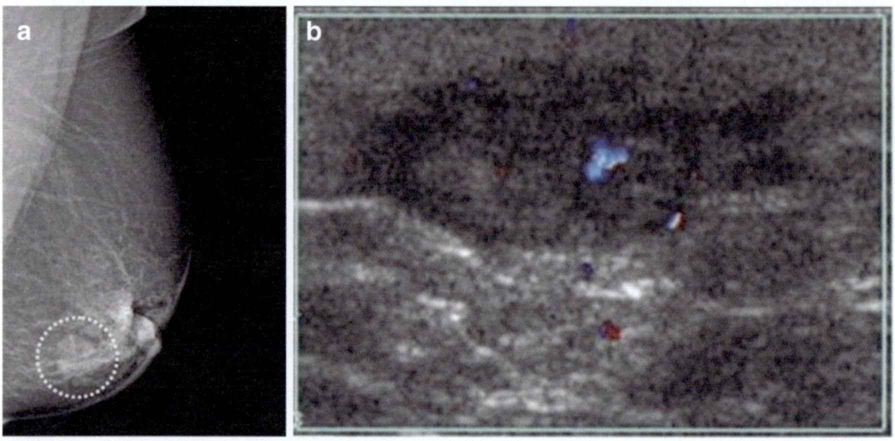

Fig. 2.17 Malignancy mimicking scar tissue on imaging
Left MLO mammogram image indicates nipple retraction and a region of architectural distortion, which contrasts with the rest of the breast being fatty tissue. Corresponding Color Doppler ultrasound imaging shows central feeding vessels and irregular shaped hypoechoic mass, indicative of malignancy

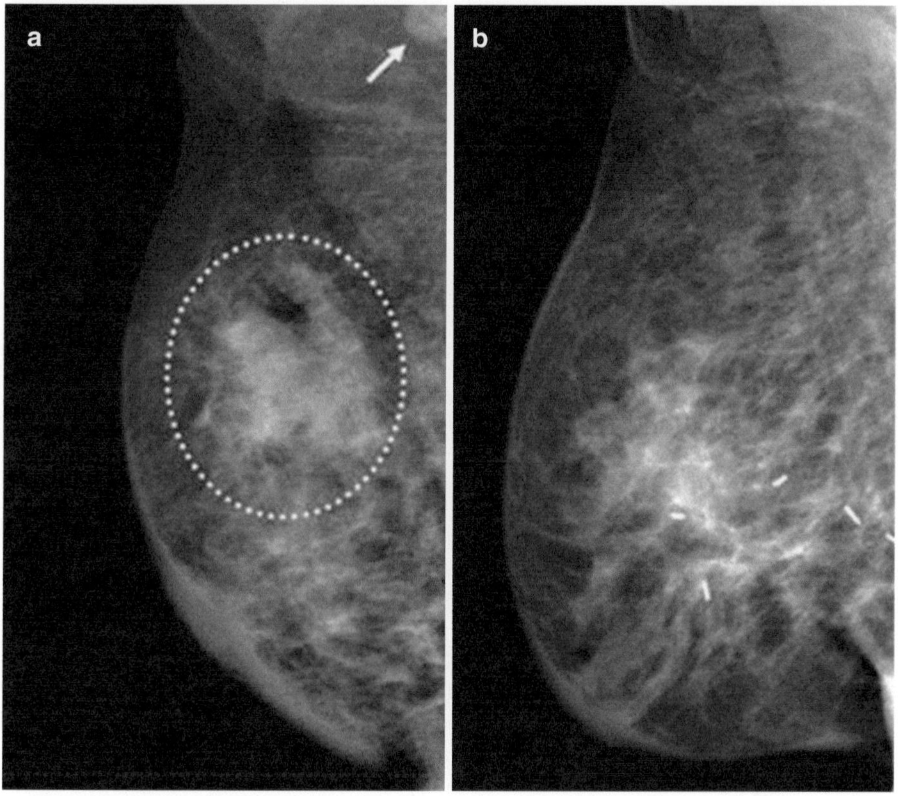

Fig. 2.18 Inflammatory breast cancer vs. post-surgical changes on mammography
Right MLO mammogram image (left) indicates a region of increased density and a large reactive node in the axillary region. Overlying skin also appears markedly thickened. Patient was diagnosed with inflammatory breast cancer
Right MLO mammogram image (right) post-surgery shows internal surgical staples present and overall enlarged breast volume in comparison to pre-surgical imaging, indicative of breast edema. Histology is suggested for confirmation thereof

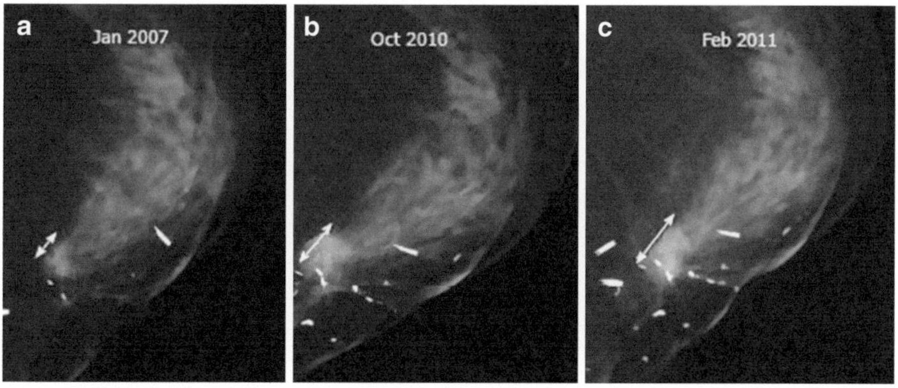

Fig. 2.19 Post-surgical calcifications on mammography
Left CC mammogram image over a 5-year period shows process of post-surgical calcifications forming over time and localized organization of the site of surgical excision [22]

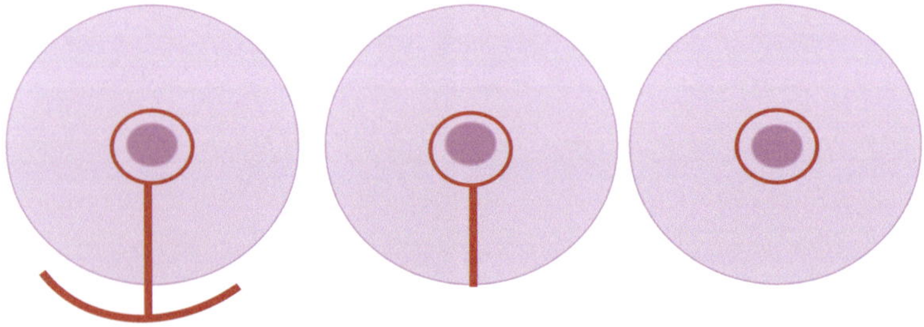

Fig. 2.20 Three most common forms of breast reduction incision used

2.6.3 Following a Mastopexy/Breast Reduction

There are various patterns of skin incisions noted following breast reduction surgery. The three most common patterns are stated below as seen in Fig. 2.20:

(a) Wise pattern, or inverted T scar or anchor scar, leaves a periareolar scar, a vertical scar in the midline of the inferior mammary, and a curvilinear scar along the inframammary fold (see Fig. 2.23).
(b) Vertical scar techniques leave a periareolar scar and a vertical scar along the midline of the lower hemisphere of the breast. The resulting scar has a lollipop-shaped appearance.
(c) Periareolar technique leaves a periareolar scar [20, 21].

Most common mammographic findings after reduction mammoplasty include parenchymal redistribution, elevation of the nipple, areolar thickening and periareolar dermal calcifications and skin thickening from scar tissue. Another characteristic finding is a retroareolar fibrotic band from the transposed flap, which can be seen extending to the repositioned NAC, parallel to the skin contour. It likely represents scarring associated with the vascular pedicle. Parenchymal redistribution occurs in 90% of cases and can be seen at mammography and MR imaging.

Typical mammographic findings in the traditional inverted T scar or Wise pattern include a downward shift of the ductal and fibroglandular tissue, as seen on the mediolateral view, and linear scar between the nipple and inframammary fold that accounts for the frequent finding of skin thickening or keloids and dermal calcifications along the inframammary fold (see Figs. 2.21, 2.22, 2.23, 2.24, and 2.25) [20, 21].

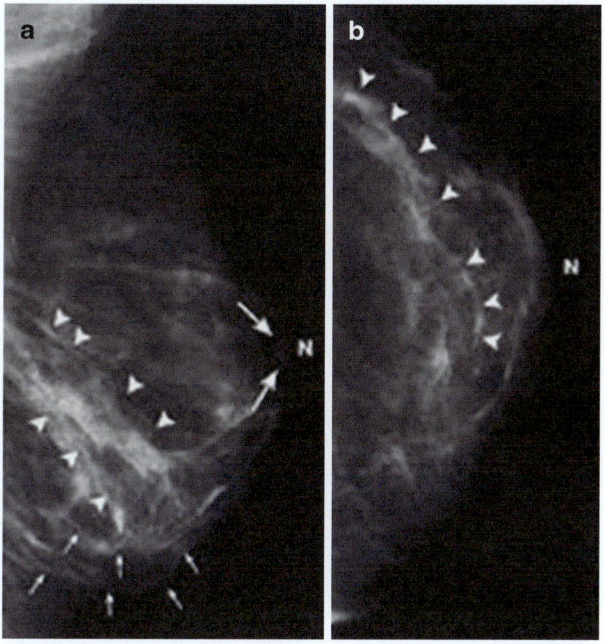

Fig. 2.21 Mammogram appearance of breast reduction surgery
Typical post-surgical appearance of the breast following breast reduction surgery, with swirling appearance of the glandular tissue [22]

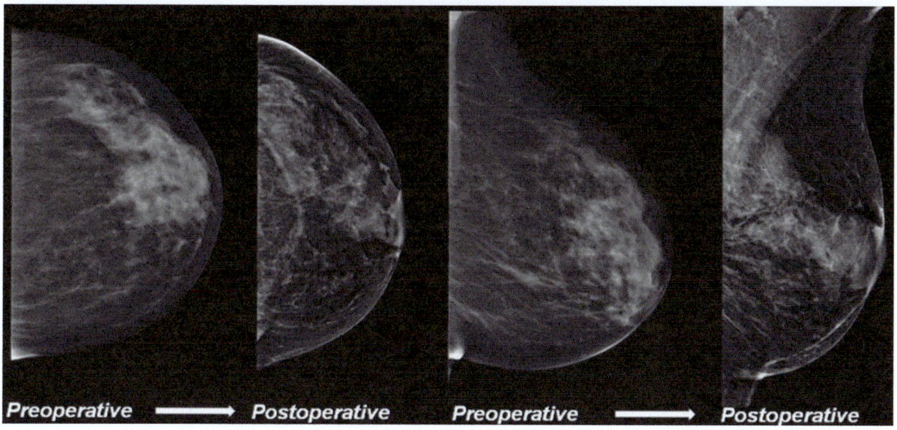

Fig. 2.22 Mammogram demonstrating the Lejour technique
Normal postoperative findings (Lejour technique). Preoperative and postoperative mammograms are shown for comparison. Mammographic findings after reduction mammoplasty include parenchymal redistribution, elevation of the nipple, areolar thickening, and inferior vertically oriented skin thickening from scar tissue [23]

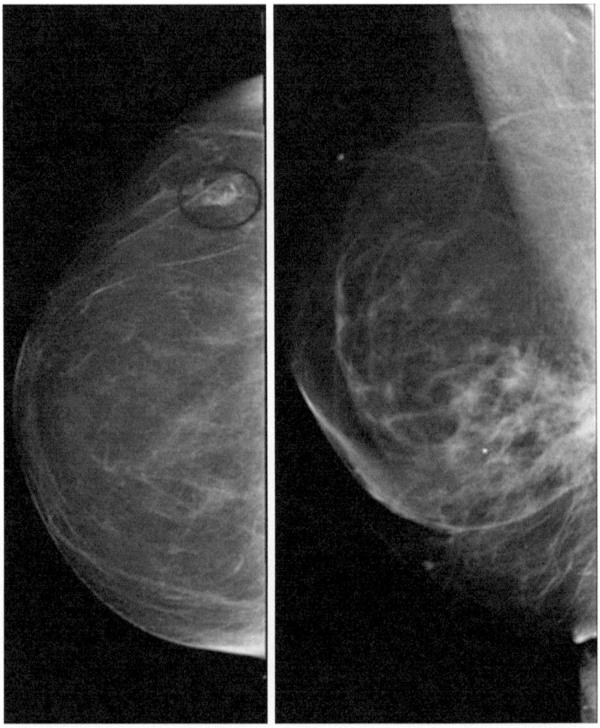

Fig. 2.23 Normal postoperative findings (Wise pattern)
Mammogram of the right breast shows a downward shift of the ductal and fibroglandular tissue and linear scar between the nipple and inframammary fold, as seen on the mediolateral view. Asymmetric density (circle) with lucent area and curvilinear calcifications is seen in outer quadrant in CC view and is related to fat necrosis [23]

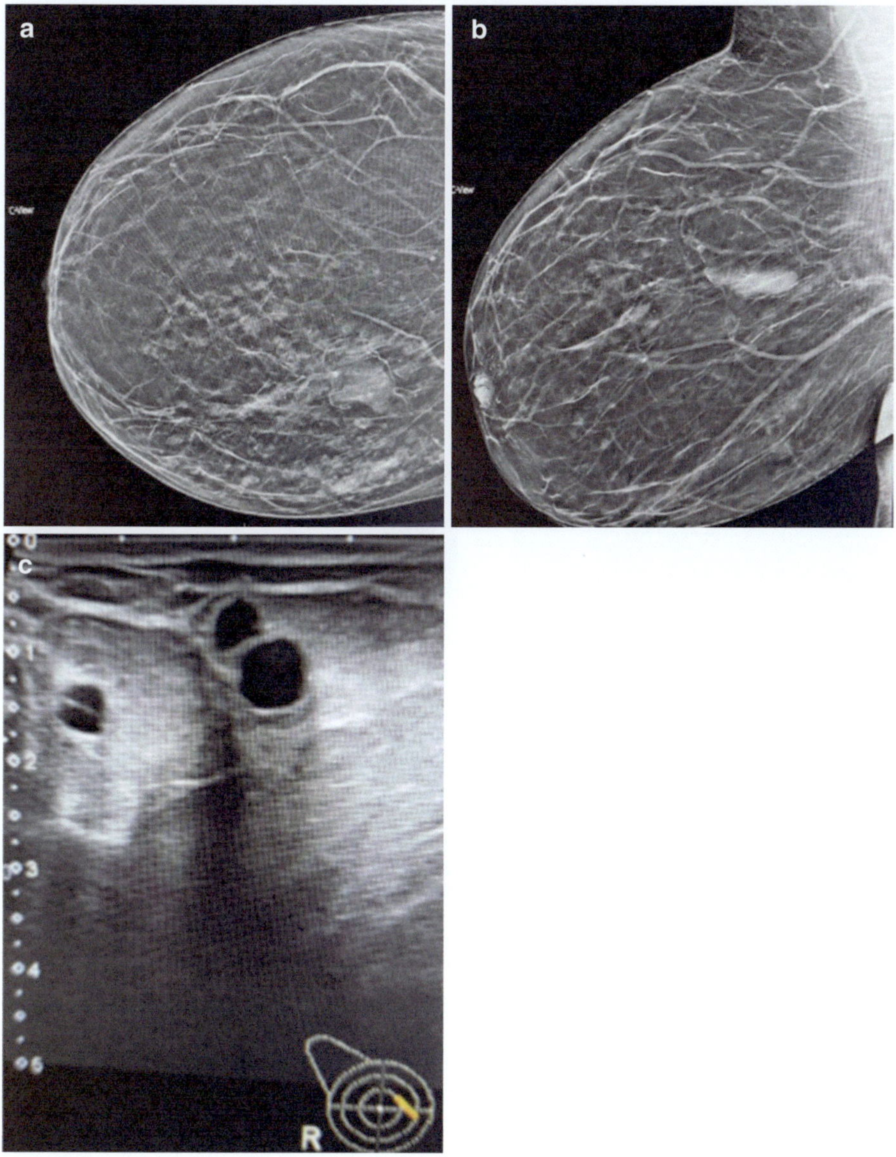

Fig. 2.24 Imaging demonstrating eggshell rim calcifications
37-year-old woman with history of reduction mammoplasty. Mediolateral oblique mammograms (**a**) reveal focal well-circumscribed radiolucency with rim calcification
Gray-scale sonogram (**b**, **c**) reveals cystic masses with internal echoes and rim calcification. Findings are consistent with benign oil cyst

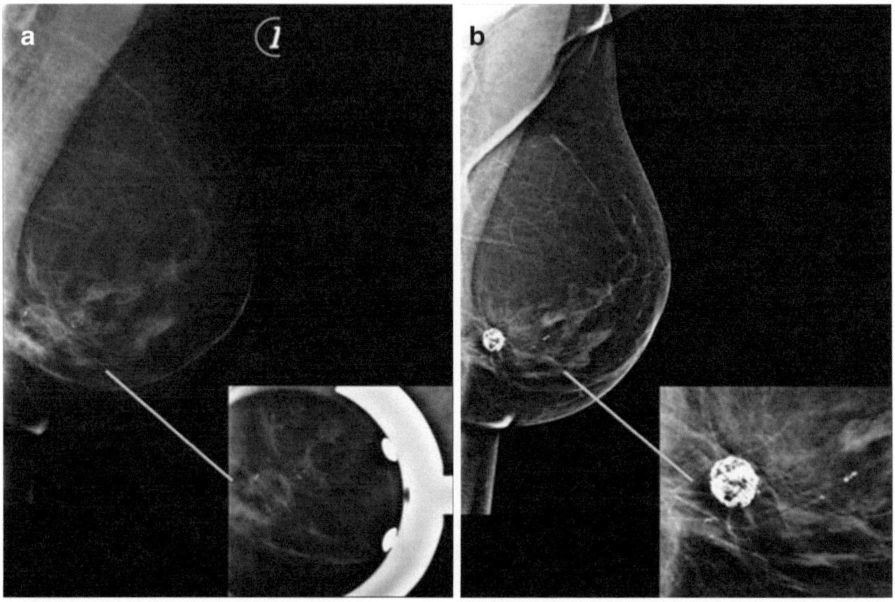

Fig. 2.25 Progressive fat necrosis on mammogram
58-year-old woman with history of reduction mammoplasty (Wise pattern). Mammogram shows downward shift of the ductal and fibro glandular tissue and linear scar between the nipple and inframammary fold, as seen on the mediolateral view. In (**a**) lucent areas and stippled curvilinear and peripheral calcifications are shown in the inferior quadrant. Mammogram obtained 4 years after (**b**) shows coarse calcifications and calcified lipid cyst compatible with progressing fat necrosis

2.7 B3 Lesion

Breast lesions of uncertain malignant potential (B3) are frequently diagnosed in the era of breast cancer (BC) screening and their management is controversial. They are generally removed surgically, but some international organizations and guidelines for breast research suggest follow-up care alone or, more recently, propose vacuum-assisted excision (VAE). The risk of upgrading to BC is known, but very little data exist on its role as a risk factor for future BC development. The B3 lesions included flat epithelial atypia (FEA), atypical ductal hyperplasia (ADH), lobular intraepithelial neoplasia (LIN), atypical papillary lesions (PLs), and radial scars (RSs) [10, 14, 24, 25].

Breast lesions of uncertain malignant potential (B3) are frequently diagnosed in the era of breast cancer (BC) screening and their management is controversial (see Fig. 2.26). They are generally removed surgically, but some international organizations and guidelines for breast research suggest follow-up care alone or,

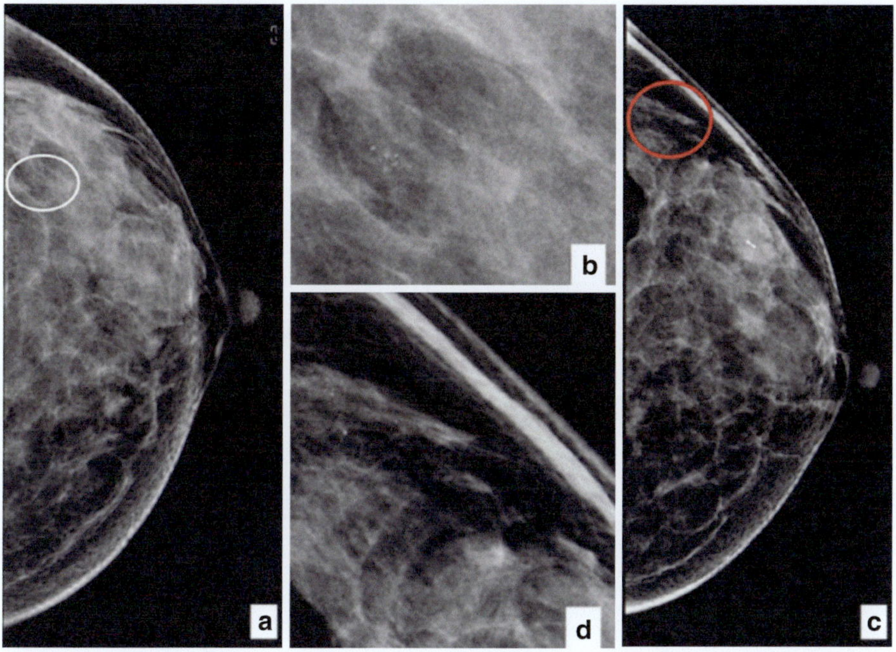

Fig. 2.26 Imaging of a B3 lesion
Figure 2.26 refers to a 49-year-old patient with a cluster of microcalcificaitons in the upper outer quadrant of the left breast (**a**) CC left view highlighting microcalcifications with white circle (**b**) Magnification view shows new formation of microcalcifications 3-year post-vacuum biopsy (**c**) CC left view highlighting calcifications with red circle, subsequent biopsy confirmed presence of DCIS [25]

more recently, propose vacuum-assisted excision (VAE). The risk of upgrading to BC is known, but very little data exist on its role as a risk factor for future BC development.

The histologic reports after biopsy with a diagnosis of a B3 lesion include flat epithelial atypia (FEA), atypical ductal hyperplasia (ADH) (see Fig. 2.27), atypical lobular hyperplasia (LIN1), and classic-type lobular carcinoma in situ (LIN2), that in the subsequent text will be collectively referred to as LIN, phyllodes tumors (PTs), papillary lesions (PLs), radial scars (RSs), and a group of rare histologic subtypes (mucocele-like lesions, myofibroblastoma, spindle cell proliferation) [10, 14, 24, 25].

Recent guidelines published by a number of breast societies suggest that high-risk women should undergo an annual mammogram examination with an additional breast MRI, or breast US or contrast-enhanced mammography in the case of contra-indication to MRI or if MRI is not readily available [10, 14, 24, 25].

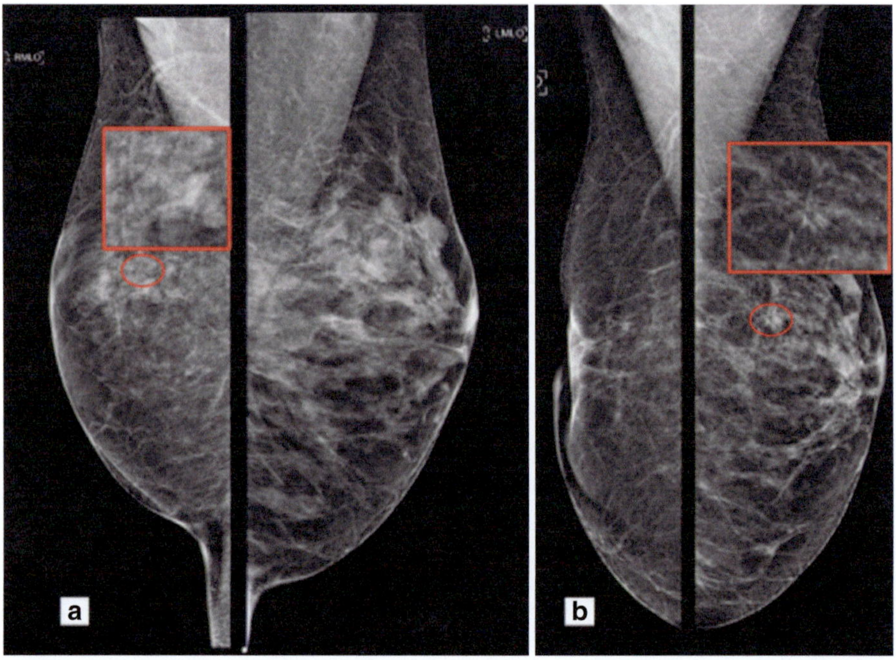

Fig. 2.27 Atypical ductal hyperplasia vs. invasive ductal carcinoma on mammography
Figure above of a 56-year-old patient with

(**a**) cluster of microcalcifications in the upper outer quadrant of the right breast, initially diagnosed as ADH, surgical excision followed

(**b**) 5 years later, developed architectural distortion in the same area of previous surgery, which was confirmed with subsequent biopsy as IDC [26]

It is known that after a diagnosis of ADH, and especially of LIN, the risk of developing BC is increased in both breasts and not just at the site of the B3 lesion. This result at least suggests that not only ADH, atypical PLs, and LIN, but also FEA represents a generic marker of BC risk that is not limited to the side of initial diagnosis.

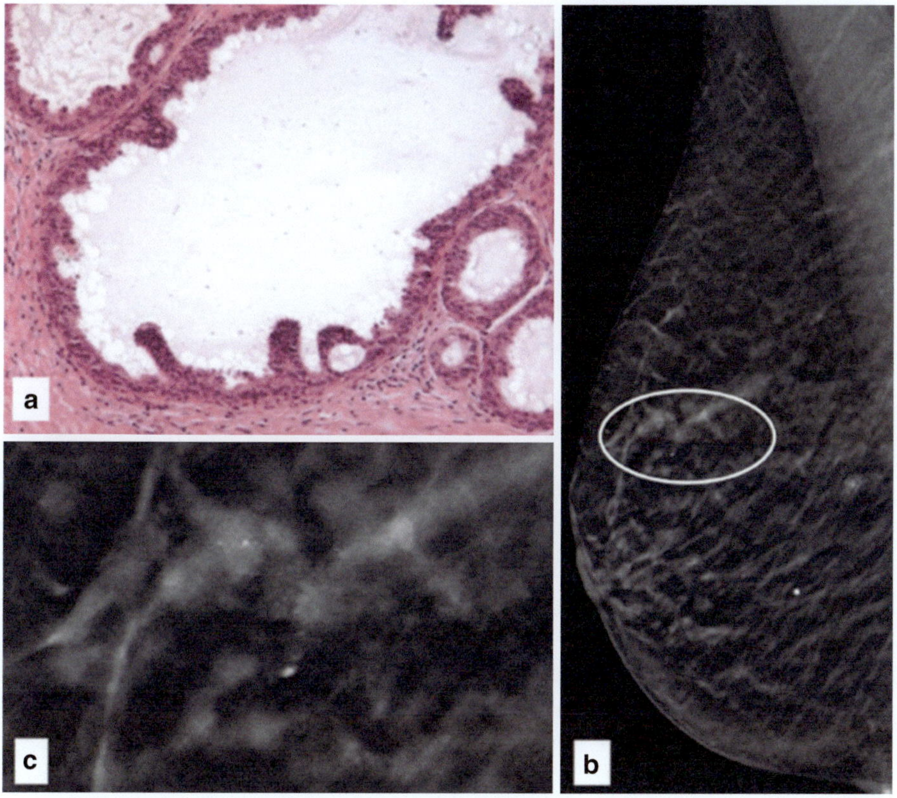

Fig. 2.28 Histological and mammographic appearance of ADH [26]

It is suggested that B3 lesions should be surgically removed and that a clinical and radiological follow-up with a yearly bilateral mammogram and US scan of the breast should be proposed for at least 5 years (see Figs. 2.28, 2.29, and 2.30). This approach may possibly translate to earlier diagnosis of BC among patients with previous B3 lesion excision, with clear clinical benefits for these patients [10, 14, 24, 25].

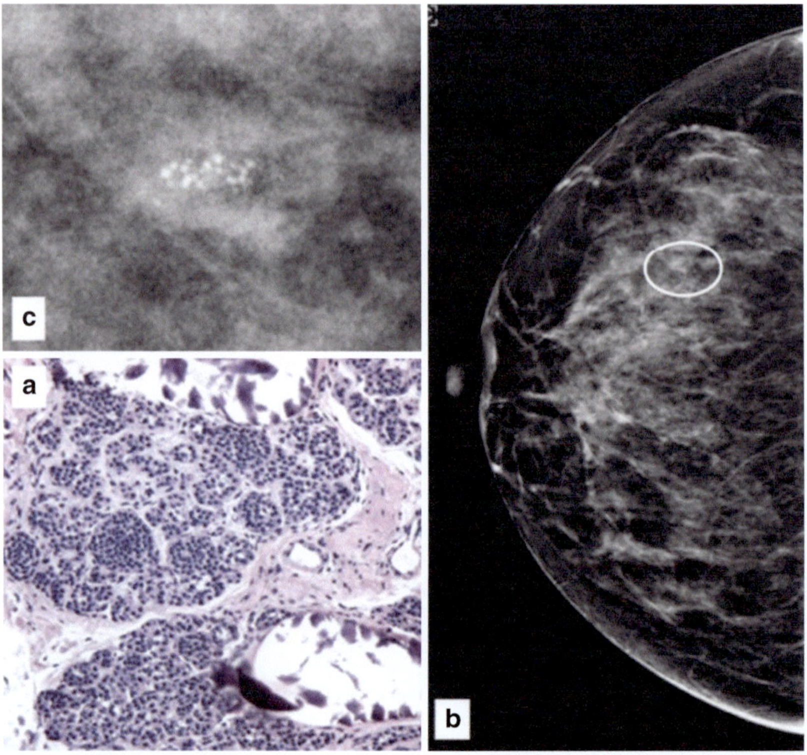

Fig. 2.29 Lobular intraepithelial neoplasia [25]

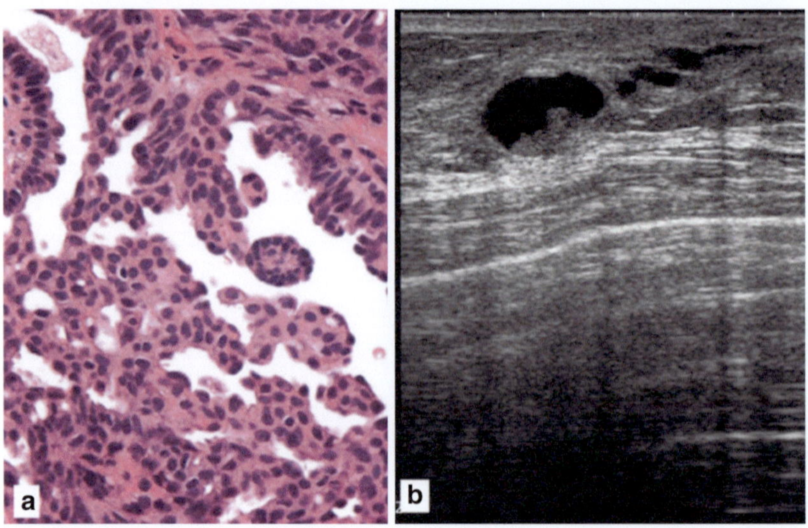

Fig. 2.30 Atypical papillary lesions [25]

2.8 Mondor's Disease

Mondor's disease of the breast (MDB) is an uncommon and benign disorder. Thrombophlebitis of the anterior chest wall's subcutaneous venous network is its defining feature. It was thoroughly documented by French surgeon Henri Mondor, who published a case series in 1939 that detailed the condition. In 50–60% of instances, no cause is discovered (primary disease); however in 40–50% of cases, certain augmenting variables may exist. Underdiagnosis occurs due to the disease's rarity and the lack of precise diagnostic criteria. In rare cases, the presence of MDB has led to the discovery of an underlying breast cancer [27, 28].

The prevalence of MDB is unknown due to its rarity and a lack of awareness of clinical signs.

MDB is considered idiopathic in 50–60% of instances. In 40–50% of situations, a favorable factor may exist. Many case reports indicate a link between local trauma (e.g., hard exercise, tight brassiere, or direct damage) and the start of the visible cord (see Fig. 2.31).

In a retrospective examination of 652 female patients who had cosmetic breast surgery, Goldman and Wollina discovered three MDB instances. Catania et al. identified eight MDB cases related to breast cancer among 68 MD cases [27, 28].

There are a few references to MDB during pregnancy. The clinical appearance is nonspecific, and physiological hypercoagulability is unlikely to be the cause of MDB production. Neoplasms, excessive sexual activity, trauma, or abstinence can all cause penile lesions. MD of the axilla, also known as axillary web syndrome, has been reported following axillary surgery. The only clinical symptom of MDB is an acute, generally painful, cord-like induration in the chest wall area, which is the patient's primary complaint. The diagnosis is made based on medical history and physical examination [27, 28].

Depending on the troublesome vein, the induration topography may vary. The thoracoepigastric vein is the most prevalent site of the lesion, followed by the lateral

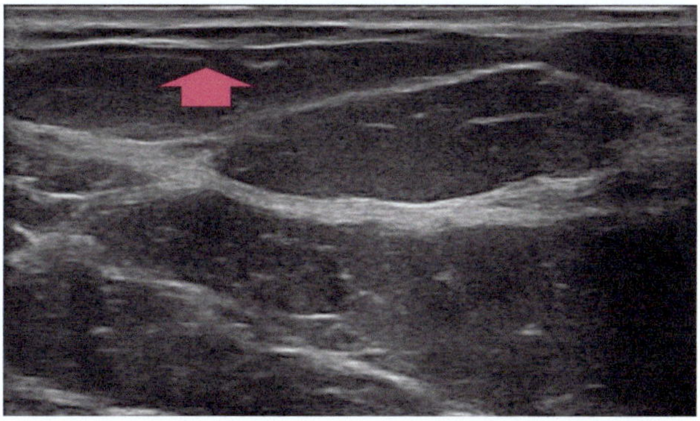

Fig. 2.31 Thrombus formation associated with Mondor's disease on ultrasound
Additional use of Color Doppler would demonstrate intravenous thrombus formation within the breast tissue's subcutaneous layer, coinciding with the clinically evident induration on the skin

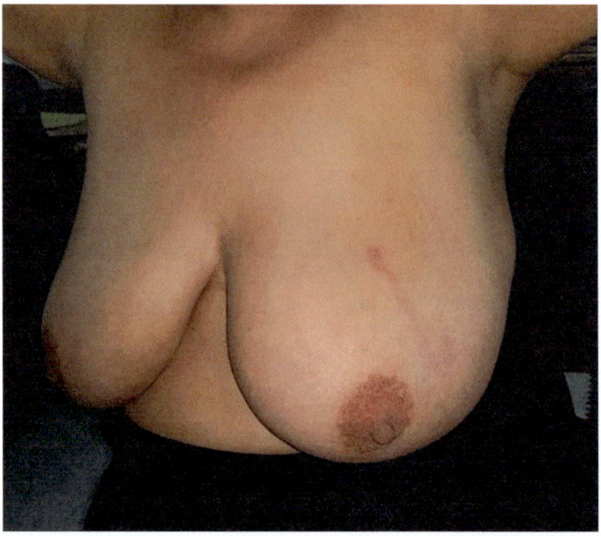

Fig. 2.32 Clinical appearance of Mondor's disease
Clinical examination confirms cord-like induration and skin erythema along the venous thrombus [27, 28]

thoracic vein and superior epigastric vein. When the clinical presentation is inconclusive, an ultrasound may be necessary. It exhibits incompressible tubular forms with anechoic or hypoechoic properties (see Fig. 2.32). Color Doppler can even be used in the absence of a flow signal within the vein [27, 28].

Mammography is used to determine the cause rather than confirm the diagnosis. In reality, because the link between MDB and breast cancer has been estimated at roughly 4% (1.8% in Herman's series and 12.7% in Catania's), mammography should be explored in both genders. There has been evidence linking MDB to breast cancer in male individuals. Magnetic resonance imaging and other imaging modalities are not suggested for assessing MDB and may result in excessive health care costs [27, 28].

MDB is typically a spontaneously regressive condition that resolves between 4 and 8 weeks, with no specific therapy required. First-line treatment includes warm compresses, painkillers, and nonsteroidal anti-inflammatory medications, as well as avoiding aggravating clothing or activities. The majority of lesions will cure on their own and require no additional treatment. However, in certain cases, the cord-like induration might be felt for months.

MDB is a self-limited condition that resolves spontaneously with no sequela. However, patients should be educated on the importance of follow-up [27, 28].

2.9 Conclusion

In conclusion, Chap. 2 has provided an in-depth exploration of benign breast diseases, encompassing a wide range of conditions that may affect individuals across different stages of life. Each section has delved into the most encountered benign pathologies, such as fibrocystic breast disease, fibroadenoma, gynecomastia, benign phyllodes tumors, and benign hyperplasia. For each condition, we have examined their pathophysiology and histopathology, discussed how they appear on clinical imaging, and considered appropriate treatment and management options.

Understanding these benign conditions is essential for accurate diagnosis and to prevent unnecessary anxiety, as they often present with similar symptoms to malignant conditions. This chapter has underscored the importance of distinguishing benign from malignant pathologies through careful imaging, histological analysis, and patient assessment. Additionally, we reviewed the changes that may occur in breast tissue following treatment or surgery, emphasizing the need for ongoing monitoring and follow-up care. The knowledge of benign breast disease forms a crucial foundation for mammographers, equipping them with the expertise needed to contribute meaningfully to patient care and support the accurate diagnosis and management of breast pathology.

References

1. Fornage BD. Local and regional staging of invasive breast cancer with sonography: 25 years of practice at MD Anderson Cancer Center. Oncologist. 2014;19(1):5–15.
2. Doi K. Computer-aided diagnosis in medical imaging: historical review, current status and future potential. Comput Med Imaging Graph. 2007;31(4–5):198–211.
3. Da Costa D, Taddese A, Cure ML, Gerson D, Poppiti R Jr, Esserman LE. Common and unusual diseases of the nipple-areolar complex. Radiographics. 2007;27(Suppl 1):S65–77.
4. Burnside ES, Sickles EA, Bassett LW, Rubin DL, Lee CH, Ikeda DM, et al. The ACR BI-RADS experience: learning from history. J Am Coll Radiol. 2009;6(12):851–60.
5. Fatima. KMMKS. Fibrocystic breast disease. Statpearls; 2023
6. Shetty MK. Breast cancer screening and diagnosis. Springer; 2014.
7. Stavros AT, Thickman D, Rapp CL, Dennis MA, Parker SH, Sisney GA. Solid breast nodules: use of sonography to distinguish between benign and malignant lesions. Radiology. 1995;196(1):123–34.
8. van Rensburg MJ. Application of ultrasound characteristics in the accurate prediction of benign versus malignant solid breast nodules. University of Johannesburg; 2011.
9. Berg WA, Sechtin AG, Marques H, Zhang Z. Cystic breast masses and the ACRIN 6666 experience. Radiol Clin North Am. 2010;48(5):931–87.
10. Dennis MA, Parker SH, Klaus AJ, Stavros AT, Kaske TI, Clark SB. Breast biopsy avoidance: the value of normal mammograms and normal sonograms in the setting of a palpable lump. Radiology. 2001;219(1):186–91.
11. Ehteshami Bejnordi B, Mullooly M, Pfeiffer RM, Fan S, Vacek PM, Weaver DL, et al. Using deep convolutional neural networks to identify and classify tumor-associated stroma in diagnostic breast biopsies. Mod Pathol. 2018;31(10):1502–12.
12. Berg WA, Leung K. In: Hooley D, Davis E, editors. Diagnostic imaging: breast. 3rd ed. Philadelphia: Elsevier; 2019.
13. Berg WA, Gutierrez L, NessAiver MS, Carter WB, Bhargavan M, Lewis RS, et al. Diagnostic accuracy of mammography, clinical examination, US, and MR imaging in preoperative assessment of breast cancer. Radiology. 2004;233(3):830–49.
14. Berg WA, Campassi C, Langenberg P, Sexton MJ. Breast imaging reporting and data system: inter- and intraobserver variability in feature analysis and final assessment. AJR Am J Roentgenol. 2000;174(6):1769–77.
15. Swerdloff RS, Ng JC. Gynecomastia: etiology, diagnosis, and treatment. Endotext. 2023;

16. Kao L, Bulkin Y, Fineberg S, Montgomery L, Koenigsberg T. A case report: lobular carcinoma in situ in a male patient with subsequent invasive ductal carcinoma identified on screening breast MRI. J Cancer. 2012;3:226–30.
17. Telli ML, Horst KC, Guardino AE, Dirbas FM, Carlson RW. Phyllodes tumors of the breast: natural history, diagnosis, and treatment. J Natl Compr Cancer Netw. 2007;5(3):324–30.
18. Kalambo M, Adrada BE, Adeyefa MM, Krishnamurthy S, Hess K, Carkaci S, et al. Phyllodes tumor of the breast: ultrasound-pathology correlation. AJR Am J Roentgenol. 2018;210(4):W173–W9.
19. Mishra SP, Tiwary SK, Mishra M, Khanna AK. [Retracted] Phyllodes tumor of breast: a review article. Int Sch Res Notices. 2013;2013(1):361469.
20. Yi A, Kim HH, Shin HJ, Huh MO, Ahn SD, Seo BK. Radiation-induced complications after breast cancer radiation therapy: a pictorial review of multimodality imaging findings. Korean J Radiol. 2009;10(5):496–507.
21. Monticciolo DL, Newell MS, Moy L, Niell B, Monsees B, Sickles EA. Breast cancer screening in women at higher-than-average risk: recommendations from the ACR. J Am Coll Radiol. 2018;15(3 Pt A):408–14.
22. Ram S, Dietsche E. Post-operative imaging surveillance of breast cancer patients status post lumpectomy with BioZorb implant placement. J Radiol Case Rep. 2021;15(2):7.
23. Plaza Loma S, Rodríguez de Diego Y, Villacastín Ruiz ME, Pintado Garrido R, Ginés Santiago A. In: Herrero MH, editor. Reduction mammoplasty: what radiologists should know. European Soceity of Radiology; 2016.
24. Kalac N, Ozkan B, Bayiz H, Dursun AB, Demirag F. Breast tuberculosis. Breast. 2002;11(4):346–9.
25. Bellini C, Nori Cucchiari J, Di Naro F, De Benedetto D, Bicchierai G, Franconeri A, et al. Breast lesions of uncertain malignant potential (B3) and the risk of breast cancer development: a long-term follow-up study. Cancers (Basel). 2023;15(13)
26. Nicosia L, Latronico A, Addante F, De Santis R, Bozzini AC, Montesano M, et al. Atypical ductal hyperplasia after vacuum-assisted breast biopsy: can we reduce the upgrade to breast cancer to an acceptable rate? Diagnostics (Basel). 2021;11(6)
27. Ben Hamida K, Ghalleb M, Triki A, Jebir I, Makhlouf R, Touinsi H. Mondor's disease of the breast: a case series. J Med Case Rep. 2021;15(1):188.
28. Aulick. KMRHBNF. Mondor disease. Statpearls; 2023

Malignant Diseases of the Breast

3

Contents

K. Malherbe, *A Mammographers Guide: Radiological and Histopathological Guidelines*, https://doi.org/10.1007/978-3-031-84667-0_3

3.1 Atypical Breast Hyperplasia

Atypical hyperplasia of the breast is defined as aberrant epithelial proliferative breast lesions that are neither subjectively nor quantitatively abnormal enough to be diagnosed as cancer in situ. These lesions can appear in both male and female breast tissues; however they are uncommon and arise as an accidental discovery in male gynecomastia cases. This chapter will discuss atypical hyperplasia of both the ductal and lobular forms of the female breast. Both of these lesions are classified as premalignant or high risk for progressing to more advanced neoplasia [1–5].

Atypical ductal hyperplasia (ADH) is a reasonably frequent lesion, estimated to occur in 5% to 20% of breast biopsies. Although not carcinoma, it is classed as a high-risk precursor lesion because of its relationship with and possible progression to ductal carcinoma [2, 3, 5, 6].

3.1.1 Histopathology

Page et al. established criteria for both atypical ductal hyperplasia (ADH) and atypical lobular hyperplasia (ALH).

ADH is defined as an unusual monomorphic epithelial population of luminal origin in the breast that falls between normal/usual hyperplasia and low-grade ductal carcinoma in situ (DCIS) on the intraductal proliferative lesion spectrum (see

Fig. 3.32). ADH will exhibit some of the characteristics of DCIS without meeting all of the criteria for low-grade DCIS. Low-grade DCIS has cribriform gaps with polarized lumens made up of extremely monotonous cells with fine chromatin arranged in a solid, cribriform, or micropapillary pattern.

When the following architectural and cytologic requirements are met, size can be used to distinguish ADH from low-grade DCIS. Low-grade DCIS requires complete involvement [2, 3, 5, 6].

3.1.2 Differential Diagnosis

When examining suspected ADH or ALH, it is crucial to assess typical ductal hyperplasia, ductal carcinoma in situ, lobular carcinoma in situ, and flat epithelial atypia, with the most important distinction being whether a lesion is ADH or low-grade DCIS. These distinctions can be made based on the histologic findings described above, with the caveat that in some challenging situations, particularly problematic borderline lesions may be classified as "ADH bordering on DCIS" or "ADH suspicious for DCIS" [2, 3, 5, 6].

3.1.3 Prognosis

Atypical ductal hyperplasia (ADH) is a reasonably frequent lesion, estimated to occur in 5% to 20% of breast biopsies. Although it is not carcinoma, it is considered a high-risk precursor lesion since it is associated with and has the potential to advance to ductal carcinoma in situ (DCIS) or invasive carcinoma.

Atypical lobular hyperplasia (ALH), like ADH, is another high-risk breast lesion that has been linked to a four- to five-fold greater lifetime chance of developing breast cancer in either the ipsilateral or contralateral breast [2, 3, 5, 6].

3.1.4 Treatment/Management

Atypical hyperplasia lesions are premalignant. Many experts believe that the patient should have a thorough surgical excision to rule out malignancy and prevent advanced neoplasia from developing if a breast biopsy reveals it. Surgical excision for core biopsies demonstrating ADH is considered standard of care. However, ALH may be an accidental finding in tiny biopsies, and surgical excision of these lesions remains controversial. In general, excision is suggested for high-risk patients. Lower-risk patients with no family history of breast cancer, BRCA1 or BRCA2 mutations, solitary lesions, or a lower BI-RADS score may benefit from surveillance and/or pharmacological therapy with estrogen receptor modulators. Patients should be advised to undergo short-term follow-up with increased mammography frequency [2, 3, 5, 6].

ADH is classified as a premalignant, high-risk lesion, whereas ALH is just a high-risk lesion. Either can be detected in conjunction with or on the perimeter of a more advanced lesion; thus, it is critical to recognize that atypical hyperplasia discovered during a biopsy may not correctly represent the larger lesion. Upgrade on surgical excision after atypical hyperplasia is discovered on biopsy ranges from 10% to 30%, with cases of atypical hyperplasia suspected for DCIS having a greater rate of upgrade following excision. Studies have failed to produce reliable, independent markers of which atypical hyperplasia lesions are linked to more aggressive entities such as high-grade DCIS or invasive malignancy [2, 3, 5, 6].

It is crucial to highlight that while surgical removal following the detection of atypical hyperplasia in a core biopsy is generally deemed appropriate, there is considerable controversy about how to manage high-risk lesions in specific circumstances. Proper management will include discussing all considerations with the patient, including a review of current treatment methods and guidelines, patient risk factors, meticulous radiologic/pathologic correlation, and the overall clinical picture (see Figs. 3.1, 3.2, and 3.3) [2, 3, 5, 6].

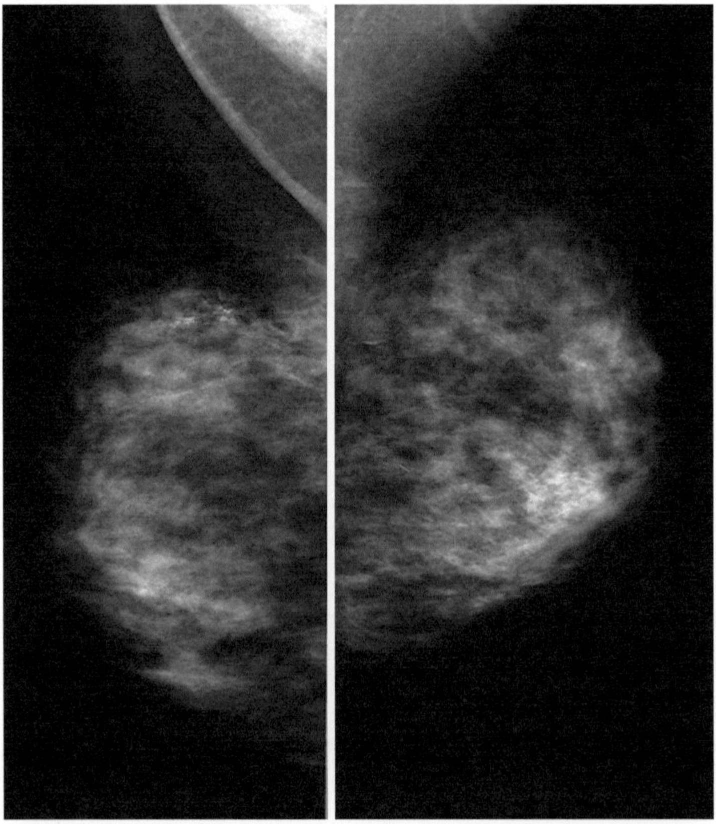

Fig. 3.1 High-risk lesions on mammography
Patient with ACR Type D tissue, presented with cluster of pleomorphic microcalcifications in the upper outer quadrant of the right breast. Histology confirmed the presence of DCIS

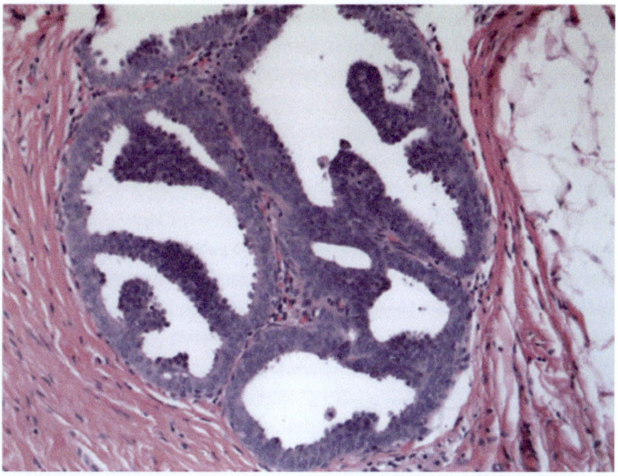

Fig. 3.2 Atypical ductal hyperplasia
ADH with cribiform and micropapillary growth pattern [3, 7]

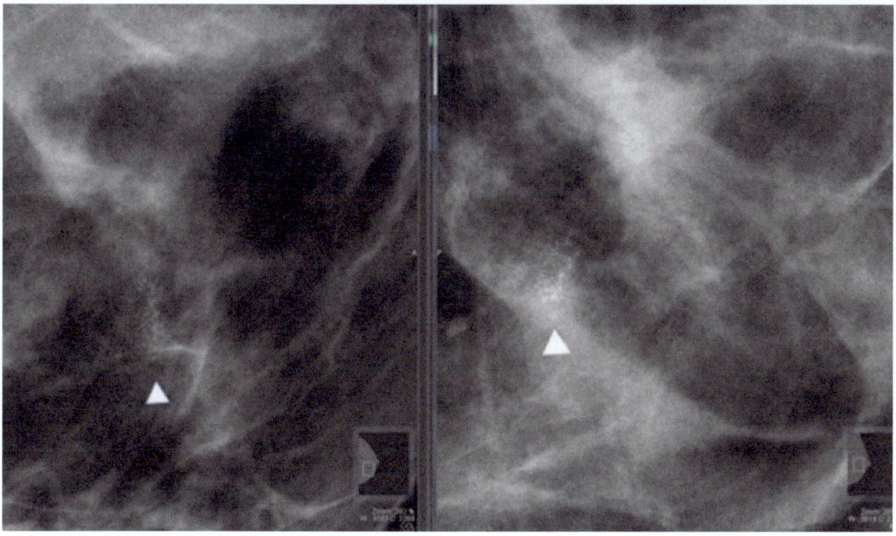

Fig. 3.3 Magnification mammography views
Figure demonstrating a cluster of pleomorphic microcalcifications confirmed with histology as atypical ductal hyperplasia [3, 7]

3.2 Ductal Carcinoma

3.2.1 Introduction

The progression from normal breast tissue to ductal cancer in situ is uncertain. Some people with DCIS have a hereditary susceptibility, particularly BRCA1 and BRCA2 mutations.

Ductal carcinoma in situ has a risk of up to 88 per 100,000 women aged 50–64 years old.

Other risk factors influence the progression of DCIS to invasive breast cancer. The risk of acquiring invasive breast cancer increases as a woman ages from birth to death by 12.3%. Increased estrogen exposure may also raise the chance of getting breast cancer. Postmenopausal women who utilize hormone replacement treatment are more likely to develop breast cancer [8–17].

Ductal carcinoma in situ (DCIS) is a clonal proliferation of epithelial cells in the breast ductal-lobular unit, restricted to the myoepithelial cell layer. It distinguishes it from invasive breast cancer. DCIS is characterized by architecture features, nuclear grade, and necrosis, with five major patterns. In micropapillary DCIS, proliferating cells produce club-shaped tufts that extend into the duct lumen and lack a fibrovascular core. Papillary DCIS causes cells to grow around fibrovascular centers. The cells in solid DCIS fill and dilate the duct. DCIS frequently exhibits many architectural patterns. Micropapillary, cribiform, and papillary DCIS are classified as low-grade lesions. DCIS with solid or comedo characteristics are high-grade lesions with a higher risk of developing into invasive cancer [8–17].

DC is categorized into low, intermediate, and high nuclear grades. Low-grade DC has uniform cells, inconspicuous nucleoli, while high-grade DC has large cells, prominent nucleoli, and frequent mitosis. Intermediate-grade DC has mild-to-moderate changes. High-grade DC increases risk of invasive breast carcinoma [8–17].

3.2.2 Pathophysiology and Histopathology

Ductal carcinoma in situ (DCIS) is a malignant, clonal proliferation of cells that grow within the breast's basement membrane-bound structures and show no signs of invasion into the surrounding stroma. Where mammographic breast screening is not undertaken, DCIS accounts for roughly 5% of breast cancers, but within screening programs, it accounts for approximately 20–25% of these tumors. However, it is now well understood that DCIS is a diverse group of lesions, clinically, radiologically, morphologically, and genetically. This heterogeneity complicates the pathologist's function in macroscopic specimen management, microscopic diagnosis, and prognostic feature assessment [8–17].

DCIS's microscopic variability has resulted in the establishment of several classification systems. Historically, DCIS was classified based on the architectural pattern of proliferation, which included comedo, cribriform, micropapillary, solid, and mixed subtypes. This classification system provides some insight into the expected amount of disease; for example, micropapillary DCIS is more likely to be multiquadrant (71%) than comedo-type disease (8%) [15]. Comedo-type DCIS presents most typically mammographically, whereas cribriform disease is more commonly detected symptomatically in some studies [8–17].

High-grade DCIS is created by massive, pleomorphic cells, frequently with many conspicuous nucleoli (see Fig. 3.4). The size of the nuclei in comparison to

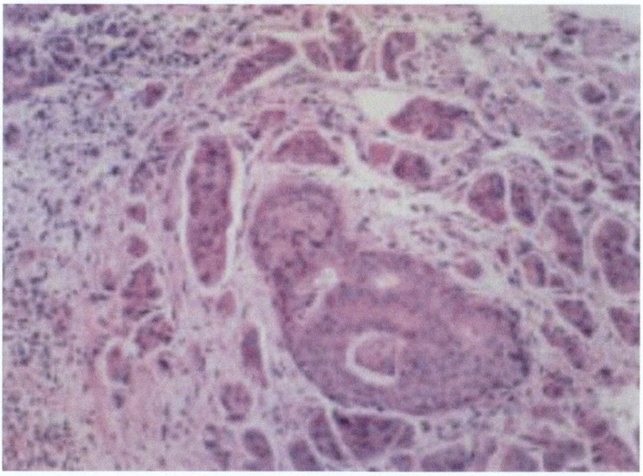

Fig. 3.4 Ductal carcinoma. The histological slide shows high-grade ductal carcinoma

surrounding normal cells, which are often normal epithelial or red blood cells, is especially useful in classification. However, comedo necrosis can occur in conjunction with other architectural patterns (for example, cribriform DCIS). The term "comedo DCIS" is extensively used in historical series, however it does not assign a specific grade or architecture to the lesion, and there is no agreement in the literature on the degree of central necrosis required, thus its repeatability as a DCIS category is doubtful [8–17].

3.2.3 Clinical Evaluation and Imaging

Screening mammography is the most common way to detect ductal carcinoma in situ, which typically does not manifest with a palpable tumor. A histologic diagnosis can be obtained with an image-guided core needle biopsy of the suspected region. Core needle biopsy samples more tissue than fine needle aspiration, allowing the pathologist to establish whether the breast cancer is invasive or noninvasive (DCIS). DCIS has traditionally been characterized architecturally as comedo, cribriform, micropapillary, papillary, or solid. Even core needle biopsy has limitations [8–17]. When a core needle biopsy confirms DCIS, there is a 10–20% probability that the excisional surgical material may have invasive cancer. Screening mammograms detect 90% of all occurrences of DCIS. Furthermore, if the patient presented with a worrisome lesion on screening mammography, diagnostic mammography is required to describe the ipsilateral disease and rule out bilateral illness (see Figs. 3.5 and 3.6). A screening mammography shows two views of the breast and is sensitive but not specific for breast cancer. Clustered microcalcification in mammograms is a typical finding in DCIS. Calcifications associated with malignancy are often smaller (0.1 to 1 mm in diameter) and grouped [8–17].

Microcalcifications with linear branching patterns or segmental pleomorphic calcifications are particularly suspicious for DCIS. When problematic calcifications

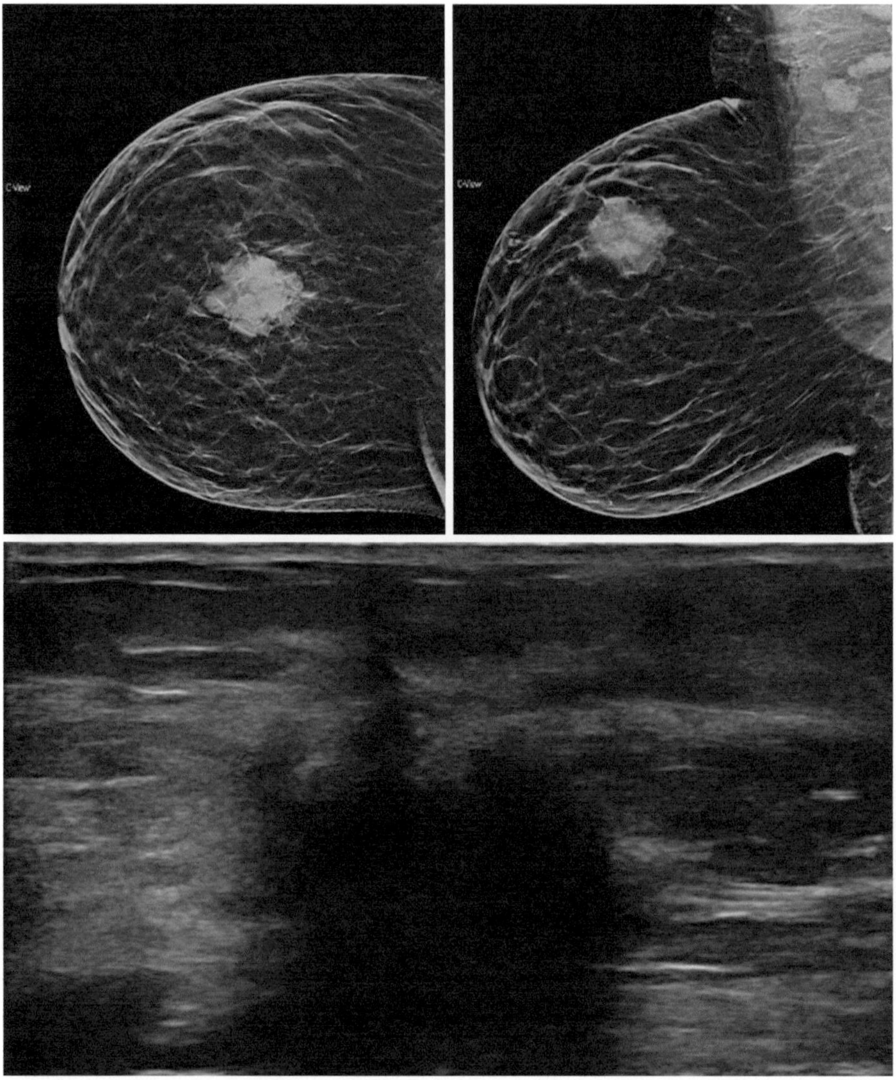

Fig. 3.5 BIRADS Category 4C
Invasive ductal carcinoma seen on CC and MLO view of the left breast as an irregular-shaped high-density mass with spiculated margins
Ultrasound image also confirms and irregular mass with angular margins and posterior acoustic shadowing

are detected on screening mammography, diagnostic mammography is required, which includes more cuts and information necessary for surgical planning [8–17].

Image-guided core needle biopsy performed on the area of suspicion will provide a histologic diagnosis. Core needle biopsy will allow for more tissue to be sampled compared to fine needle aspiration; this will allow the pathologist to

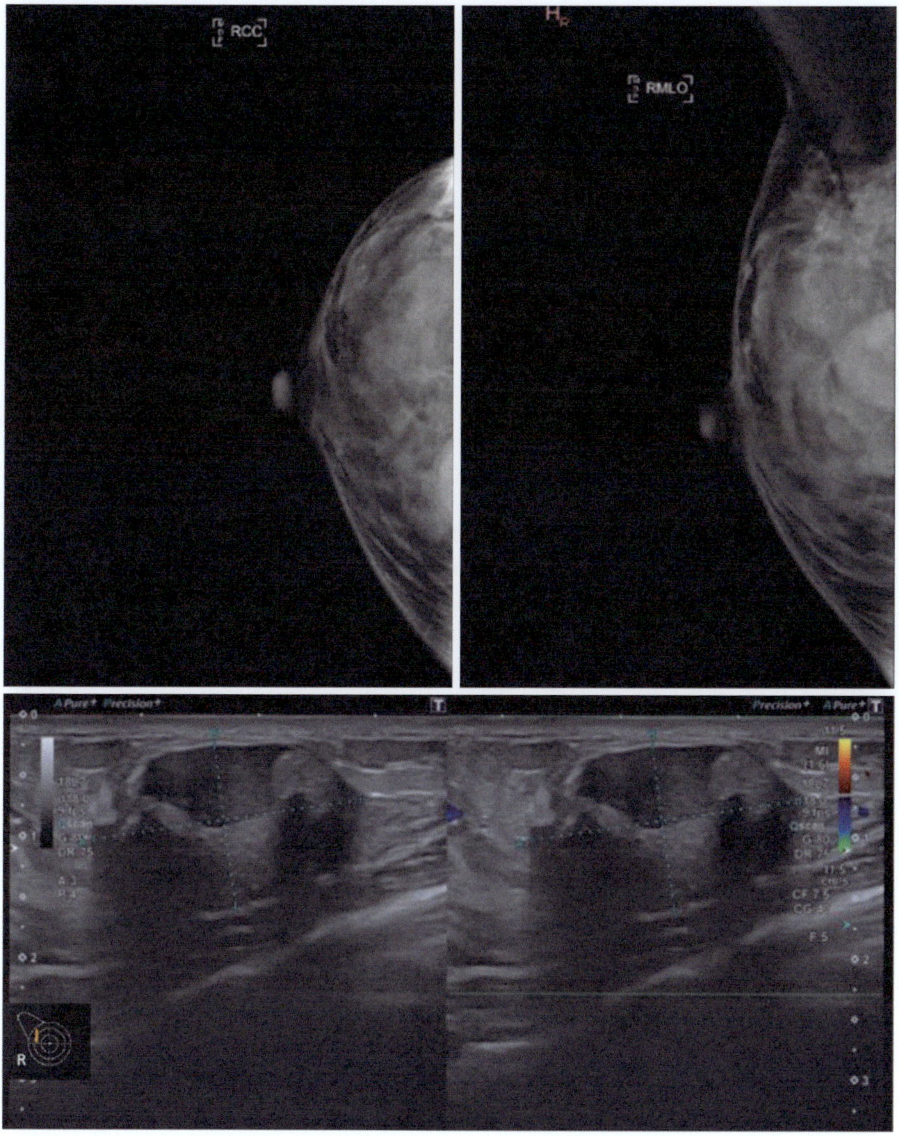

Fig. 3.6 Multimodality imaging of triple negative breast cancer
The right breast ACR type D, Ill defined, poorly circumscribed density
B-mode ultrasound confirms an irregular hypoechoic complex cystic mass
CT scan shows multiple heterogeneous masses in the right breast. Smaller ill-defined areas of enhancement in the superior and inferior medial aspect of the right breast
Breast MRI also demonstrates an irregular mass in the right breast at 12 o'clock
Nonmass enhancement noted in the subareolar aspect of the right breast, which suggests involvement of the right retroareolar fibroglandular tissue

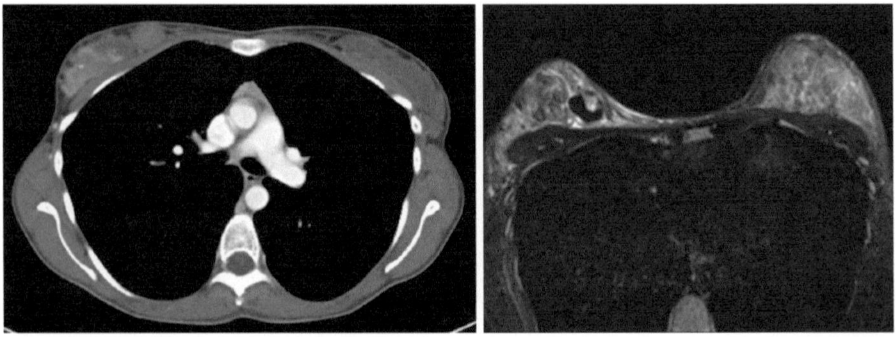

Fig. 3.6 (continued)

determine if breast cancer is invasive or noninvasive (DCIS). Classically, DCIS has been classified architecturally as comedo, cribriform, micropapillary, papillary, or solid. Of note, even core needle biopsy has limitations. When core needle biopsy reveals DCIS, there is still a 10% to 20% chance that the final excisional surgical specimen will contain invasive carcinoma [8–17].

Tissue biopsy should also be used to determine hormone receptor status, namely estrogen receptor (ER), progesterone receptor (PR), and human epidermal growth factor receptor 2 (HER-2) status. Although new receptors are being discovered and explored, these three are critical to detect. Specific endocrine treatment modalities can be used to further lower risk in people with ER/PR/HER-2 receptor positive [8–17].

3.2.4 Treatment and Management

Treatment for ductal carcinoma in situ is multimodal and involves a combination of surgery, radiation therapy, and hormone therapy that is personalized to the patient's specific diagnosis and preferences [8–17].

DCIS surgical treatment options include breast-conserving surgery followed by radiation or a simple mastectomy. It is critical to underline that both treatment options have comparable long-term survival rates. Breast-conserving therapy (BCT) with partial mastectomy and radiation is widely suggested because it is a less medically invasive method. BCT is not recommended for patients with multicentric illness, an extensive disease with little surviving breast tissue for cosmesis, or those who cannot get radiation therapy. Mastectomy is curative in 98% of patients with DCIS, regardless of tumor size or grade [8–17].

DCIS is noninvasive by definition, and axillary lymph node involvement is uncommon; therefore, sentinel lymph node (SLN) biopsy is not recommended during breast-conserving surgery. Data from the NSABP B24 trials show that axillary recurrence rates were 0.36 per 1000 patient years of follow-up, regardless of treatment (BCT vs. mastectomy). An SLN biopsy should be investigated for patients undergoing mastectomy for DCIS since an occult invasive breast cancer may be discovered, and an SLN biopsy is frequently not achievable after a mastectomy [8–17].

Endocrine therapy is the primary medical intervention for DCIS in patients with ER-positive or PR-positive DCIS. Data show that 5 years of endocrine therapy in the appropriate patient reduces the likelihood of both ipsilateral and contralateral illness. Tratuzumab may benefit HER-2-positive patients [8–17].

3.3 Ductal Carcinoma In situ

3.3.1 Introduction

Detecting, diagnosing, and managing ductal carcinoma in situ (DCIS), a non-obligate precursor to invasive cancer, remains a source of debate. DCIS incidence increased with the expansion of screening mammography programs in the 1980s and 1990s, and it is regarded as a primary cause of overdiagnosis and overtreatment. Pathologists face challenges in diagnosing and classifying DCIS due to undersampling and interobserver heterogeneity.

Understanding the path from normal breast tissue to DCIS and, eventually, to invasive cancer is hampered by a lack of natural history data, despite several hypothesized evolutionary models of DCIS start and progression. Although radiologists are familiar with DCIS's typical presentation as asymptomatic calcifications on mammography, the increased pool of modalities, sophisticated imaging techniques, and image analytics have found numerous possible biomarkers of histopathologic features and prognosis. Nonsurgical care of DCIS, such as active surveillance, is gaining popularity as it reduces overtreatment and offers more tailored treatment options for patients [7, 11, 17–20].

3.3.2 Pathophysiology and Histopathology

DCIS refers to a diverse group of lesions that exhibit a wide range of histopathologic characteristics. The basic categorization approach is based on a three-tier nuclear grading scheme that takes into account nuclear proliferation, mitotic figures, and architecture [10]. Nuclear grade is roughly evenly split between high-grade (42%) and intermediate-grade (43%) DCIS, with a smaller proportion of low-grade DCIS (14%) [7, 11, 17–20].

The nuclear grade is one of the most important distinguishing aspects of DCIS because it is connected with disease prognosis, likelihood of progression to invasive carcinoma upon surgical excision, and eligibility for active monitoring. However, a key hurdle to clear grading is a lack of reproducible measurements, as several studies have revealed significant interobserver variability among pathologists, even when using a basic two-tier system (high versus nonhigh grade) and/or majority opinion-based ratings [7, 11, 17–20].

Nuclear grade also affects DCIS imaging manifestations, such as a higher proportion of high-grade DCIS detected on MRI versus low-grade DCIS shown on US. Several studies have found that radiomic characteristics on mammography and MRI correspond with nuclear grade. However, because nuclear grade is generally determined through pathologic examination after biopsy, predicting nuclear grade from imaging has limited clinical relevance [7, 11, 17–20].

Other key standard-of-care DCIS markers include hormone receptor status, particularly ER, and necrosis, particularly comedo-like necrosis. Around 87% of DCIS cases are ER positive. ER status is significant because it correlates with invasive recurrence and prognosis and allows for adjuvant endocrine therapy. ER status also corresponds with imaging presentation; for example, ER-negative DCIS is more likely to be apparent at US, whereas ER-positive DCIS manifests as fine pleomorphic and fine-linear branching calcifications [7, 11, 17–20].

Atypical ductal hyperplasia and low-grade DCIS have similar morphologic characteristics, but a DCIS diagnosis needs at least two completely involved ducts or a diameter of at least 2 mm [10]. As a result, a core needle biopsy sample containing only one tiny, affected duct may produce a diagnosis of atypical ductal hyperplasia, which is later upgraded to DCIS during surgical excision (Fig. 3.1). Similarly, the use of a 14-gauge automated biopsy device (vs. an 11-gauge vacuum-assisted device) and fewer biopsy samples is more likely to miss concomitant invasive cancer at the initial core biopsy, which is then upstaged to invasive cancer during surgery [7, 11, 17–20].

3.3.3 Clinical Evaluation and Imaging

DCIS is most usually detected (about 80%) as asymptomatic calcifications on mammography. Approximately half of DCIS calcifications will have fine pleomorphic morphology and a clustered distribution. Fine pleomorphic, fine-linear, or fine-linear branching calcifications are more common in high-grade DCIS and DCIS with necrosis, while round calcifications are associated with low-grade DCIS [7, 11, 17–20].

However, Breast Imaging Reporting and Data System descriptors alone are unable to distinguish between nuclear grades. Noncalcified mammographically identified DCIS occurs in roughly 10% of DCIS diagnosis, frequently appearing as a mass (67%) and less likely as a focal asymmetry (24%) or architectural distortion (15%) [7, 11, 17–20].

Although noncalcified pure DCIS has a fair prognosis, calcified DCIS with an accompanying tumor, asymmetry, or architectural deformation increases the risk of progression to invasive cancer. Finally, women with palpable DCIS have a higher risk of a noncalcified appearance (14% vs. 4% for all DCIS in one series) [7, 11, 17–20].

Despite the fact that calcifications arise frequently on mammography (see Fig. 3.7), their cause is unknown. Breast calcifications are thought to form by both passive (degenerative or dystrophic) and active (secretory or bone matrix protease)

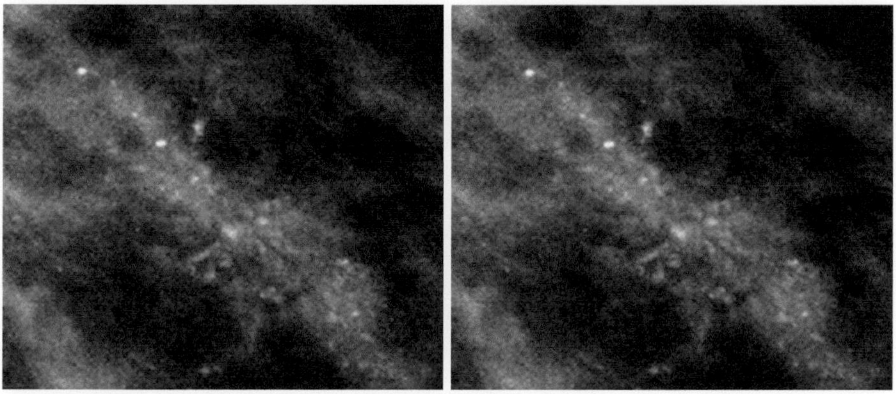

Fig. 3.7 Branch-like microcalcifications on mammography
Typical branch-like pattern of ductal carcinoma on magnified mammogram image [23]

mechanisms, with two main chemical components: calcium oxalate (type I) and calcium hydroxyapatite (type II) [7, 11, 17–20].

Type I calcifications are typically linked with benign processes, but type II calcifications are more commonly associated with malignant processes [21, 22]. Differences in the underlying physiologic genesis of calcifications are believed to explain the wide range of morphological appearances, as well as the relationship between calcification morphologic traits and distribution and DCIS nuclear grade and hormone receptor status [7, 11, 17–20].

Although screening mammography is commonly used to detect DCIS, nearly half of DCIS lesions can be diagnosed in women who undergo US. The most typical presentation is a hypoechoic irregular hypervascular mass with a parallel direction and no posterior characteristics (Fig. 3.3). Alternatively, a mass with a "pseudo microcystic" appearance, consisting of both solid and microcysts, is hypothesized to be caused by lobular distention in the terminal ductal-lobular units [7, 11, 17–20].

Ductal abnormalities such as an increase in the number of ducts due to neogenesis, ductal ectasia, or intraductal echogenic material may be present, and modest intraductal material with low-level echoes may be misdiagnosed as benign ductal ectasia [24]. For unknown reasons, ER-negative DCIS is more likely to be detected sonographically than ER-positive DCIS (61% vs. 46%, respectively) [7, 11, 17–20].

Noncalcified DCIS detection rates with US (95%) are higher than those with digital breast tomosynthesis (84%) and mammography (68%) [25]. Mammographically occult DCIS diagnosed by the US is more likely to be of lower severity (see Fig. 3.8), with less comedonecrosis and amplification of human epidermal growth factor receptor 2 [7, 11, 17–20]. This could be owing to a slower development rate that adheres to ductal anatomy and does not produce mass effect or necrosis-induced calcifications that are visible on mammography, but the source is unknown [7, 11, 17–20].

DCIS is most usually seen as nonmass enhancement on MRI, with masses or foci of enhancement appearing less frequently. Gadolinium enhances DCIS by causing

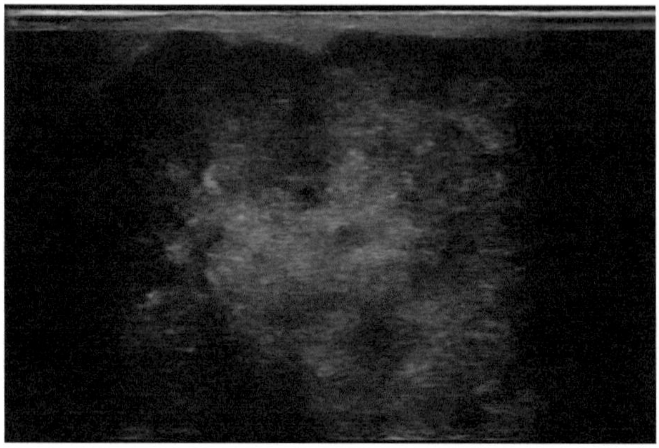

Fig. 3.8 Branch-like microcalcifications on ultrasound
High-frequency ultrasound systems of 18 MhZ or more can also illustrate calcifications within an ill-defined mass as seen in this image

vascular and basement membrane permeability within the ducts. Given its restriction to the milk ducts, it is understandable that the bulk of DCIS that manifests as nonmass enhancement (60%–80%) is segmentally or linearly distributed depending on the number of ducts and lobules involved [7, 11, 17–20].

Such distributions are likely to reflect typical DCIS proliferation, which begins with intraductal tumorigenesis and progresses to local proliferation along the ductal channel. Internal morphologic aspects have also been proposed as a possible explanation for DCIS's proliferative development pattern [7, 11, 17–20]. For example, clumped internal enhancement may reflect patchy intraluminal carcinoma cell proliferation, whereas a clustered ring may indicate a greater preference for peripheral growth and periductal stromal angiogenesis, as well as a higher rate of progression to invasive disease [7, 11, 17–20]. DCIS lesions exhibit peak contrast enhancement later than invasive tumors, with a lower proportion demonstrating delayed phase washout [7, 11, 17–20].

The MRI appearance of DCIS reflects the underlying biology and is associated with outcomes. For example, DCIS discovered by MRI is more likely to be of high nuclear grade than DCIS diagnosed by mammography. Semiquantitative MRI features can be used to discriminate DCIS nuclear grades and identify low-risk DCIS using the Van Nuys score. However, radiomics heterogeneity parameters such as low gray-level run emphasis and short run low gray-level run emphasis approached statistical significance in distinguishing high from nonhigh nuclear grade DCIS. \ AQ{Please check and edit the sentence ``Quantitative assessments of lesion\ ldots''for clarity.}Quantitative assessments of lesion size or volume [7, 11, 17–20].

Contrast-enhanced mammography is a new imaging method that is gaining popularity for applications such as assessing response to therapy, preoperative staging, and, perhaps, screening (see Fig. 3.9). Contrast-enhanced mammography may be an effective method for diagnosing and managing DCIS because it compensates for the limitations of mammography (i.e., lack of enhancement) and MRI (i.e., inability to display calcifications) [7, 11, 17–20]. Contrast-enhanced mammography, in particular, may aid to better define the extent of disease by distinguishing between calcified and noncalcified DCIS, as well as to identify occult invasive carcinoma by detecting

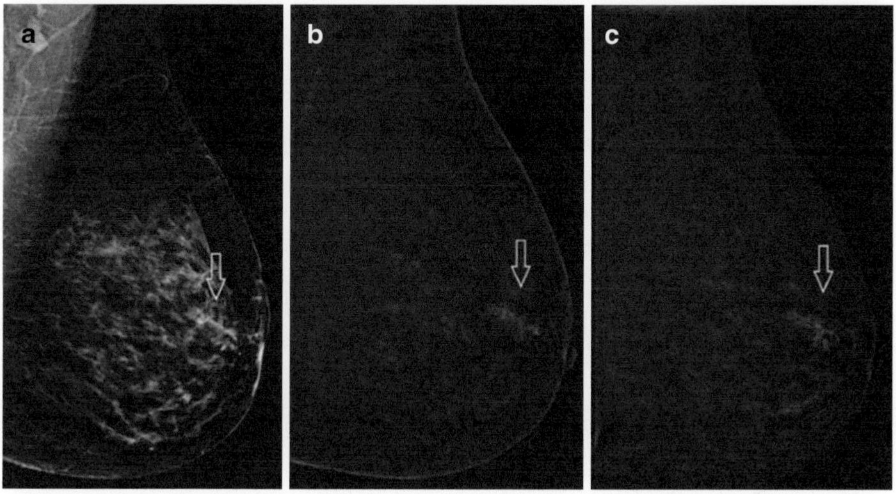

Fig. 3.9 Patient with ductal carcinoma in situ. (**a**) Low-energy mammogram demonstrates an asymmetry. (**b**) and (**c**) show early and late phases of nonmass enhancement

enhancing invasive malignancy in the presence of DCIS calcifications. Although only a small number of retrospective studies on contrast-enhanced mammography have included numerous DCIS patients so far (range, 19–37 DCIS cases), they illustrate the promise of contrast-enhanced mammography [7, 11, 17–20].

3.3.4 Treatment and Management

Because the vast majority of patients are treated after being diagnosed, there is little information available about the natural history of DCIS and the amount of overtreatment. A series of older investigations in patients with missed DCIS lesions found that roughly 25% of patients who did not get surgical excision experienced an ipsilateral invasive breast event within 15 years after diagnosis [7, 11, 17–20].

A more recent cancer registry research in women who did not have surgery after being diagnosed with DCIS found that the 15-year risk of ipsilateral invasive carcinoma was 10–20% lower. The chance of developing invasive cancer in the same breast appears to vary by lesion subtype, with nonhigh-grade (nuclear grade I or II) and hormone receptor-positive lesions having a lower risk [7, 11, 17–20].

Despite limited sample sizes and selection biases in these observational studies, available data support the notion that most patients with DCIS would not develop invasive breast cancer if they did undergo immediate surgery. The most definitive answer regarding the propensity to progress to invasive cancer, however, will result from ongoing randomized studies that are evaluating active surveillance as an alternative to immediate surgery [7, 11, 17–20].

3.4 Invasive Ductal Carcinoma

3.4.1 Introduction

Invasive ductal carcinoma (IDC), also known as infiltrating ductal carcinoma, is a kind of breast cancer that begins in the milk ducts of the breast and spreads to surrounding tissue. IDC may eventually spread (metastasize) to other parts of the body via lymph nodes or the circulation. This is referred to as metastatic breast cancer. Male breast cancer is most commonly diagnosed as invasive ductal carcinoma.

Some individuals may be diagnosed with a subtype of IDC. These diagnoses are rare, accounting for less than 5% of all breast cancers. Less prevalent kinds of IDC are:

- Medullary carcinoma.
- Metaplastic carcinoma.
- Mucinous (or colloidal) cancer.
- Papillary carcinoma.
- Tubular carcinoma [7, 11, 17–20]

3.4.2 Pathophysiology and Histopathology

Invasive ductal carcinoma (IDC) exhibits highly variable histopathological features, most commonly assessed using the modified Bloom-Richardson grading system, also referred to as the Nottingham grading system. This grading system evaluates three key components: tubule formation, nuclear pleomorphism, and mitotic count, with each component scored on a scale of 1–3, yielding a total score out of 9 [7, 11, 17–20].

Atypical cells in IDC often exhibit a size greater than twice the diameter of red blood cells, though they may appear bland, particularly in tubular carcinomas. These cells frequently contain nucleoli and may form ducts or sheets. Mitotic figures and necrosis may or may not be present. Evidence of invasion is often characterized by the presence of atypical nuclei adjacent to adipocytes, a diagnostic hallmark, and an infiltrative growth pattern, where small glands of varying sizes are embedded within a desmoplastic stroma. These glands are lined by a single layer of malignant cells [7, 11, 17–20].

Immunohistochemistry (IHC) plays a pivotal role in confirming invasive carcinoma. The absence of myoepithelial markers, such as SMMS and p63, supports the diagnosis of invasion. Prognostic markers are critical for guiding treatment decisions. Estrogen receptor (ER) positivity is observed in approximately 75% of cases, typically assessed using the Allred or Quick score. Progesterone receptor (PR) staining is more variable, and ER-negative/PR-positive tumors are exceedingly rare, occurring in less than 1% of cases, leading some to question the clinical utility of PR testing. HER2 positivity is found in 15–20% of IDC cases. Ki67, a marker of proliferation, correlates with prognosis, but its broader clinical application is limited by inconsistencies in quantification.

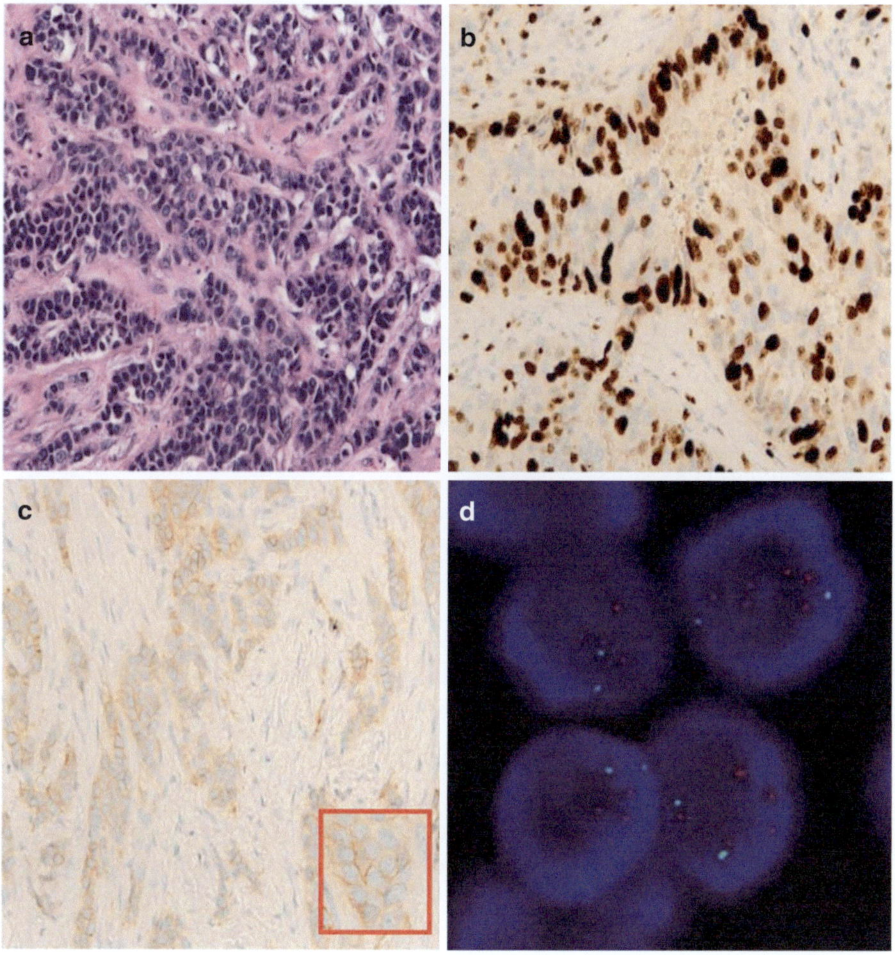

Fig. 3.10 IDC HER-2-positive histology image [26]
FISH testing of HER-2-positive breast cancer

Distinguishing invasive lobular carcinoma (ILC) from IDC often relies on E-cadherin staining (see Fig. 3.10). IDC typically shows strong membranous E-cadherin positivity, although 3–5% of high-grade IDC cases may lack this expression. Conversely, ILC is generally E-cadherin negative, though up to 15% of ILC cases may exhibit weak or incomplete staining [7, 11, 17–20].

3.4.3 Clinical Evaluation and Imaging

Invasive ductal carcinoma (IDC) may be detected incidentally on mammography before the onset of symptoms, though clinical presentations vary. Common symptoms include noticeable changes in breast shape, breast or nipple pain, nipple

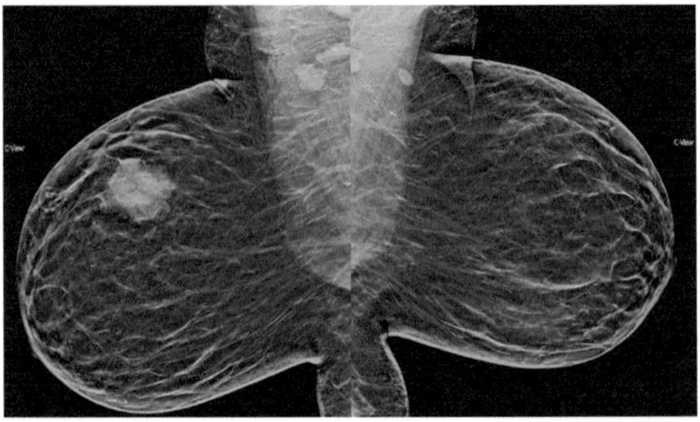

Fig. 3.11 IDC on mammogram
Right MLO demonstrating an irregular spiculated mass with the so-called tent sign. Also note enlarged lymph nodes in the right axilla

discharge, localized swelling, a palpable lump within the breast tissue, or thickening of the nipple skin. Clinically, IDC often presents as a large, immobile mass that can be palpated during a physical examination.

Mammographic findings for IDC typically include an irregular mass that may or may not exhibit calcifications. The mass is often spiculated and hyperdense, seen in 41% of grade 1 tumors and 26% of grade 3 tumors [9, 20, 27]. Circumscribed masses are more frequently observed in grade 3 tumors (36%). Microcalcifications are common, with approximately 34% of grade 1 and 37% of grade 3 tumors exhibiting them (see Fig. 3.11). The morphology of calcifications provides insight into tumor grade, with amorphous calcifications associated with low-grade IDC and pleomorphic calcifications more common in high-grade tumors [2, 28, 29].

On ultrasound, IDC appears as an ill-defined, hypoechoic mass with hyperechoic angular margins (see Fig. 3.12). Posterior acoustic shadowing is observed in 71% of grade 1 tumors, whereas posterior enhancement is more common in grade 3 tumors (45%). The mass may demonstrate ductal extension, indicative of its spread into adjacent breast parenchyma. Ultrasound also reveals a branched or spiculated pattern, with microcalcifications occasionally visible within the lesion [2, 28, 29].

Elastography, an advanced ultrasound technique, reveals increased stiffness in both the mass and surrounding tissue. This stiffness correlates with the tumor's grade, making it a useful adjunct in IDC evaluation [2, 28, 29].

Magnetic resonance imaging (MRI) provides further characterization of IDC. On T1-weighted imaging, the tumor is typically isointense to the surrounding breast parenchyma and hypointense to fat. Post-contrast T1 imaging (T1 C+ Gd) reveals an irregular or spiculated mass with characteristic ring enhancement that progresses centripetally, or nonmass enhancement (NME). Dilated veins may be seen draining the tumor. Kinetic curves from contrast uptake show early washin with a high initial enhancement ratio (IER), and the lesion often demonstrates a washout or plateau kinetic curve, seen in 76–91% of IDC cases. On T2-weighted imaging, IDC appears iso- to hypointense relative to the parenchyma, with hyperintense signals corresponding to an edematous peritumoral zone.

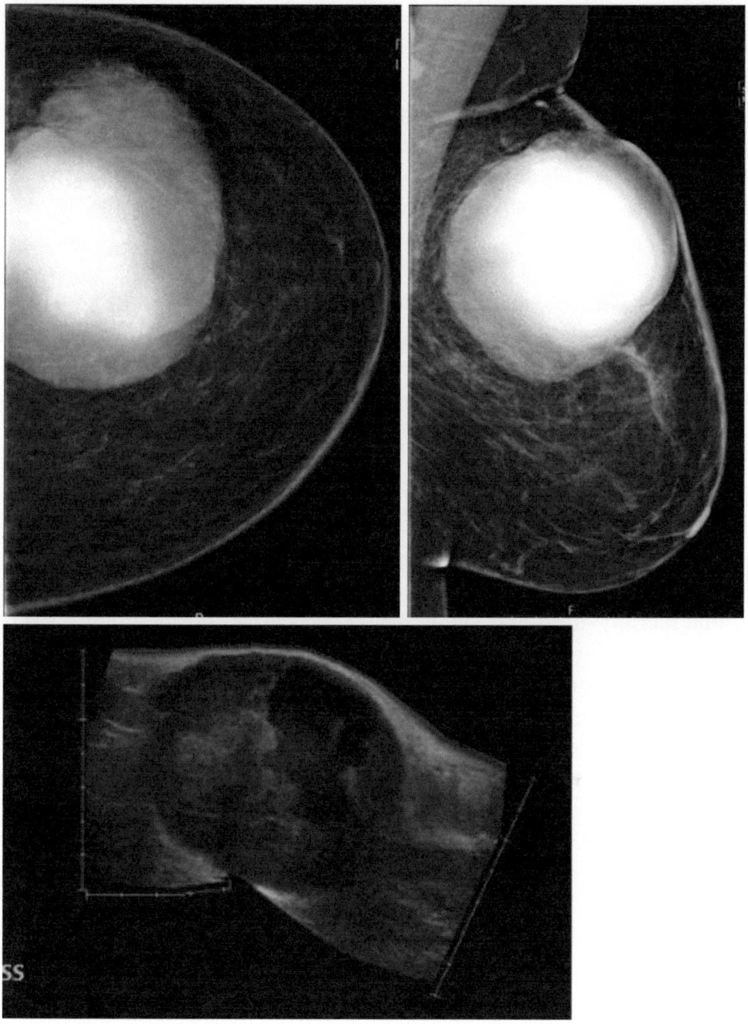

Fig. 3.12 An unusual presentation of poorly differentiated IDC as an abscess like mass. Note the use of panoramic view on B-mode ultrasound to visualize the extent of the mass

These imaging modalities, combined with clinical examination, are critical for the early detection, diagnosis, and management of IDC [2, 28, 29].

3.4.4 Treatment and Management

The treatment and management of invasive ductal carcinoma (IDC) are highly individualized, beginning with an accurate diagnosis. A multidisciplinary approach, involving breast cancer pathologists and radiologists, ensures precise determination of the tumor's characteristics, including hormone receptor status (estrogen and progesterone) and HER2 expression. This critical information guides the selection of appropriate treatments tailored to the patient's specific cancer profile [2, 28, 29].

The choice of IDC treatment depends on various factors such as the stage of the cancer, tumor size, lymph node involvement, and the patient's overall health. Since IDC can be diagnosed at any stage from I to IV, the treatment strategies can range from localized therapies to systemic approaches or a combination of both.

Surgical intervention is a cornerstone of IDC treatment, with options including lumpectomy or mastectomy. In early-stage IDC, a lumpectomy may be sufficient to excise the tumor while preserving the breast. In more advanced or late-stage cases, a mastectomy, involving removal of the entire breast, may be necessary [2, 28, 29].

Radiation therapy often follows lumpectomy to ensure the eradication of any residual cancer cells and to reduce the risk of recurrence. The use of radiation is especially crucial when breast-conserving surgery is performed.

Systemic therapies are essential in the treatment of IDC, particularly when the cancer has spread beyond the breast or there is a high risk of recurrence. Systemic treatments include:

Chemotherapy, which targets rapidly dividing cancer cells and is often employed in cases of high-risk or advanced-stage IDC [2, 28, 29].

Hormone therapy, used in patients whose tumors are hormone receptor positive, helps block or lower the levels of hormones like estrogen, which can fuel the growth of certain breast cancers [2, 28, 29].

Targeted therapies are employed in cases where tumors overexpress the HER2 protein, a growth-promoting factor. These therapies specifically target HER-2-positive cancer cells to slow their growth and progression [2, 28, 29].

The Nottingham Prognostic Index (NPI)

Is a tool used to predict the prognosis of patients following surgery for IDC. It incorporates three key factors: the size of the tumor (S), the status of the lymph nodes (N), and the tumor grade (G). The NPI is calculated using the formula: [30] = (0.2 \times S) + N + G,

where:

- S represents the size of the lesion in centimeters.
- N is the node status (0 nodes = 1, 1–3 nodes = 2, >3 nodes = 3).
- G refers to the tumor grade (scored 1 to 3).

The NPI provides insight into long-term survival outcomes:

- NPI $\leq$2.4: Excellent prognosis, with a 96% 10-year cancer-specific survival rate.
- NPI >2.4 and $\leq$ 3.4: Good prognosis, with a 93% 10-year survival.
- NPI >3.4 and $\leq$ 5.4: Moderate prognosis, with a 78% 10-year survival.
- NPI >5.4: Poor prognosis, with a 44% 10-year survival.

By combining the NPI with other clinical factors, physicians can refine treatment strategies, enhancing outcomes and tailoring therapies to each patient's unique situation.

3.5 Lobular Carcinoma and Invasive Type

3.5.1 Introduction

Invasive lobular carcinoma is the second most frequent histologic type of breast cancer, accounting for 5% to 15% of all invasive cases. It is made up of non-cohesive cells that are either scattered singly or grouped in a single-file linear pattern in the fibrous stroma. Invasive lobular carcinoma is typically accompanied with lobular cancer in situ. It is now recognized as a physiologically separate illness from the more prevalent invasive ductal carcinoma, with distinctive molecular pathogenesis. This has consequences for diagnosis and treatment. Understanding these variations is critical for developing effective management methods [1, 2, 5, 9–11, 13, 15, 18–20, 27, 28, 31–46].

Molecular studies support the idea that lobular carcinoma in situ and atypical lobular hyperplasia are non-obligate precursors to invasive cancer, not just risk indicators.

CDH1 mutations and PIK3CA genes play a significant impact in the development of lobular breast cancer [1, 2, 5, 9–11, 13, 15, 18–20, 27, 28, 31–46].

According to GLOBOCAN 2018, the global incidence of breast cancer is 46.3 per 100,000 people. In the United States, the incidence is 84.9 per 100,000 people with a death rate of 12.7 per 100,000. Breast cancer is the second leading cause of death after lung cancer. Lobular carcinoma of the breast accounts for 5–15% of all invasive breast cancers, with an average age of diagnosis 3 years higher than invasive ductal carcinoma [5]. Recent research indicated that lobular tumors are more likely to be Luminal A between 45% and 51%. These are less frequent in young (≤ 50 years) and Black women and are bigger, low grade, with less TP53 pathway abnormalities [1, 2, 5, 9–11, 13, 15, 18–20, 27, 28, 31–46].

3.5.2 Pathophysiology and Histopathology

Infiltrating lobular breast cancer has a poor rate of full pathological response (0–11%) following neoadjuvant chemotherapy. Positive resection margins during breast conservation surgery are relatively common. 17–65% of the cases require additional surgical intervention. CDH1/E-cadherin mutations are detected at rates ranging from 12% to 83%. TP53, PIK3CA, FOXA1, ZNF703, FGFR1, and BCAR4 are among the molecular variables associated with infiltrating lobular breast cancer or the progression of lobular carcinoma in situ to invasive cancer [1, 2, 5, 9–11, 13, 15, 18–20, 27, 28, 31–46].

Invasive lobular carcinomas typically present as irregular and poorly delimited tumors that are difficult to define macroscopically due to the diffuse growth pattern of the cell infiltrate. The size of the ILC is likewise impossible to determine, despite previous reports.

Invasive lobular carcinoma is characterized by a proliferation of tiny cells lacking cohesiveness. These cells might be scattered singly through fibrous connective tissue or grouped in single-file linear cords entering the stroma. The invading cords frequently form a circular pattern around regular ducts. The background architecture usually has minimal reaction from the hosts. The neoplastic cells feature round or notched ovoid nuclei and a thin rim of cytoplasm with an infrequent intracytoplasmic lumen, which frequently contains a central mucoid inclusion [1, 2, 5, 9–11, 13, 15, 18–20, 27, 28, 31–46]:

1. Several invasive lobular carcinoma variants share the cytology and development pattern of classic cases but lack cell-to-cell cohesiveness.
2. Solid type.
3. Pleomorphic lobular carcinoma.
4. Tubulo-lobular variation.
5. Alveolar variation.
6. Mixed variation.

Although the literature estimates that 80–95% of invasive lobular carcinomas are positive for estrogen receptor (ER), in current practice, classic invasive lobular carcinomas are almost always ER positive. ER-positive invasive carcinoma accounts for 70–80% of all special types. Progesterone receptor (PR) positivity is seen in 60–70% of both tumor types. HER2 overexpression and amplification are uncommon in invasive lobular carcinoma but present in some pleomorphic lobular carcinomas. Invasive lobular carcinomas rarely express p53, basal markers (keratin 14, keratin 5/6, EGFR), and myoepithelial markers (smooth muscle actin, p63) [1, 2, 5, 9–11, 13, 15, 18–20, 27, 28, 31–46].

MIB1/Ki67 labeling shows modest proliferation rates in invasive lobular carcinoma, but greater in variations. Loss of expression of E-cadherin, a cell-cell adhesion protein, is a common molecular alteration in invasive lobular carcinoma and its variants. This contributes to the discohesive nature of lobular cells (see Fig. 3.13).

Histologic grading of invasive lobular carcinomas using the Nottingham system is recommended, despite it clearly correlates with the nuclear grade. Pure lobular tumors score a 3 for tubule development; the only nuclear grade 1 lesion is histologic grade 1, although the bulk of invasive lobular carcinomas have nuclear grade 2, qualifying them for histologic grade 2. Except for few pleomorphic invasive lobular carcinomas, few tumors have histologic grade 3 [1, 2, 5, 9–11, 13, 15, 18–20, 27, 28, 31–46].

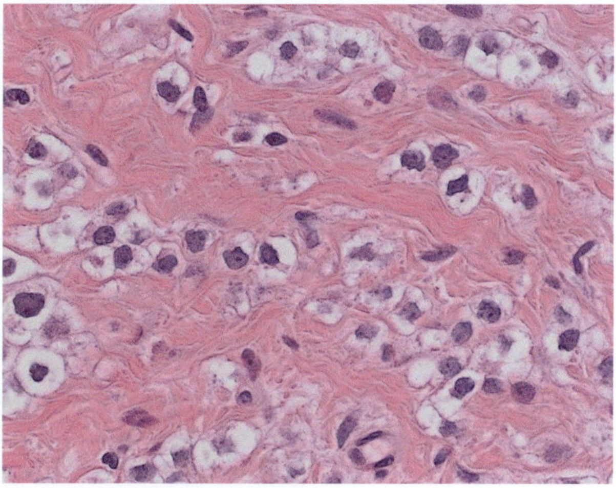

Fig. 3.13 Histopathology of invasive lobular carcinoma

3.5.3 Clinical Evaluation and Imaging

Invasive lobular carcinoma patients may present with a tumor or widespread nodules. They are also identifiable with mammographic breast screening. Invasive lobular carcinoma shares similar histological and clinical characteristics with other types of invasive breast cancer. Invasive lobular cancer is typically clinically quiet and goes undetected on mammograms or physical examinations until the illness progresses. This is due to the neoplasm's slow growth and infiltrative nature, which make early detection challenging using a mammogram [1, 2, 5, 9–11, 13, 15, 18–20, 27, 28, 31–46].

Patients in advanced stages have a palpable lump, often with a modest thickening of the nipple or an exudative scab on the skin, as well as other skin alterations such as flushing, edema, and the possibility of metastasis to the axillary or supraclavicular lymph nodes. As a result, the doctor should thoroughly examine the patient to ensure that no important information is missed.

Invasive lobular carcinomas are difficult to detect clinically and radiographically, and hence they tend to be larger upon diagnosis. They are frequently poorly defined and might be missed during fine needle aspiration and needle core biopsies due to the tumor cells' low cellularity and bland character [1, 2, 5, 9–11, 13, 15, 18–20, 27, 28, 31–46]:

- Invasive lobular carcinoma is challenging to identify via mammography, with higher false negative rates compared to other invasive malignancies (see Fig. 3.14).
- Invasive lobular cancer can appear with the following mammographic findings:
- A mass (up to 65% of cases) with uneven edges, generally hypothesized but occasionally confined.
- Architectural distortion and asymmetric focal density.

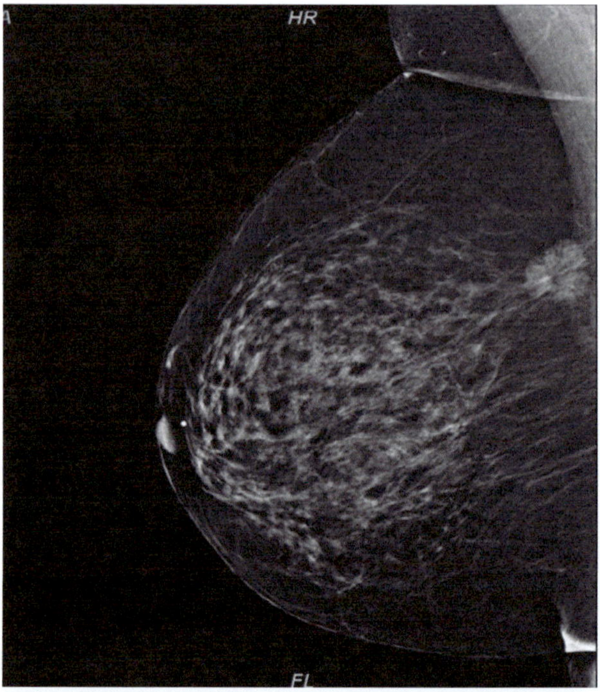

Fig. 3.14 Right MLO demonstrating a spiculated dense mass in the retromammary space (the so-called danger zone). Histology confirmed the presence of ILC

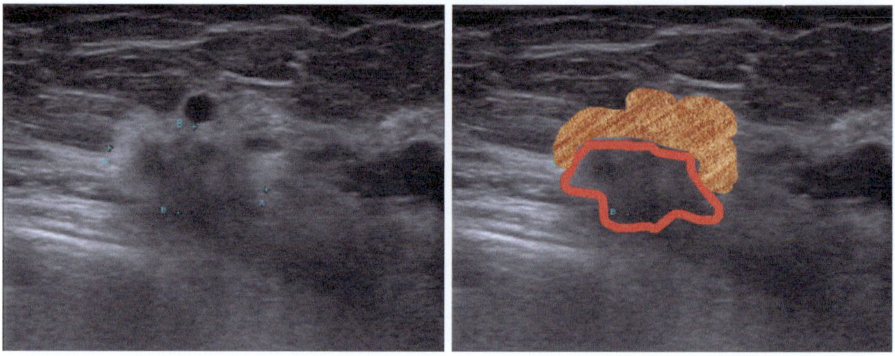

Fig. 3.15 B-mode ultrasound image of ILC
The corresponding US image of Fig. 3.14, demonstrated the typical ill-defined borders of lobular carcinoma on imaging

- Microcalcifications are uncommon (0–24%).
- In invasive lobular carcinoma, mammographic results may be normal or benign in 8–16% of cases.

Ultrasonography can reveal several manifestations of invasive lobular carcinoma (see Figs. 3.15 and 3.16), including:

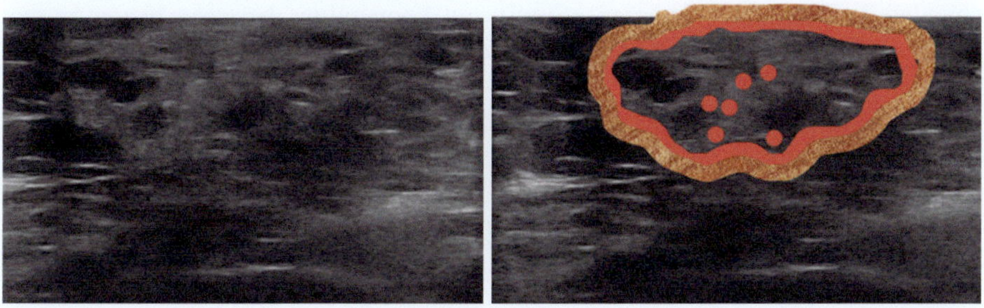

Fig. 3.16 B-mode ultrasound indicates a region of architectural distortion. Image on the right demonstrating the typical ill-defined border with a hyperechoic appearance on ultrasound

Fig. 3.17 MRI image of ILC
MRI evaluation revealed an irregular mass at 9 o'clock with relatively fast washout on kinetics. No further disease was identified on MRI

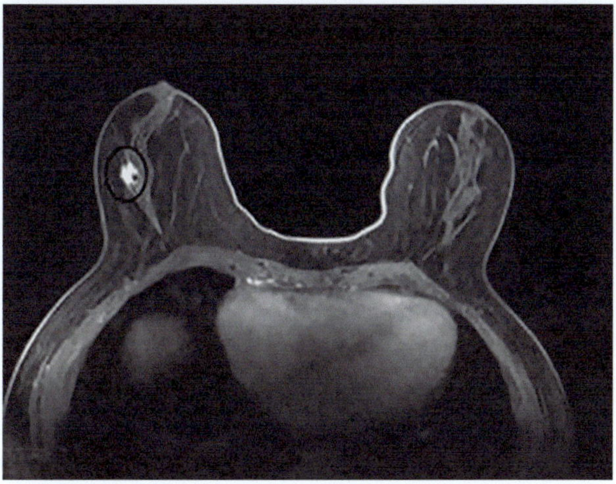

- A hypoechoic mass with uneven or unclear borders and posterior acoustic shadowing (60%).
- Shadowing with no visible bulk (15–18%).
- Mass lesions with well-defined borders (9–13%).
- Sonographically invisible (about 10%).

In one study, ultrasound screening was found to improve sensitivity and negative predictive value when used in conjunction with annual mammography in detecting breast cancer in women with a history of lobular neoplasia diagnosed after BACAF or an excisional biopsy. (sensitivity: 83%, specificity: 72%, negative predictive value: 97%) [1, 2, 5, 9–11, 13, 15, 18–20, 27, 28, 31–46].

MRI can effectively diagnose tumor margins, size, and multifocality in invasive lobular carcinoma, surpassing ultrasonography and mammography (see Fig. 3.17).

Preoperative magnetic resonance is more successful in detecting contralateral breast cancer in its early stages in older women who have positive hormone receptors. Invasive lobular carcinoma typically presents as an enhancing lump with spiculated or ill-defined borders. Significant connections between histology and MRI enhancement patterns have been found. Classic invasive lobular carcinomas with tumor cells flowing along septa are visible at MRI as enhanced septa with no dominating tumor center [1, 2, 5, 9–11, 13, 15, 18–20, 27, 28, 31–46].

3.5.4 Treatment and Management

The treatment of invasive lobular carcinomas has been a source of contention due to their probable bilaterality and multifocality. Determining the degree of invasive lobular carcinoma is crucial in selecting therapy options. The treatment is interdisciplinary, involving surgery, hormonal therapy, radiation therapy, and chemotherapy. It is a generally slow-growing cancer that can be treated over time using a variety of management options.

Mastectomy/lumpectomy is the treatment of choice for invasive lobular carcinomas in most major series, and preventive contralateral mastectomy is not uncommon. Conservative therapy for invasive lobular carcinomas is recommended if preoperative studies rule out widespread multifocal and contralateral disease. Wider negative margins are not necessary for invasive lobular cancer [1, 2, 5, 9–11, 13, 15, 18–20, 27, 28, 31–46].

Surgery and radiotherapy offer locoregional control. The lack of fibrotic response in invasive lobular carcinomas makes it challenging for surgeons and pathologists to accurately evaluate disease progression and achieve tumor-free margins during mastectomy/lumpectomy. The TNM stage at presentation determines the course of surgery, regardless of histology. Operable cancer can be treated with surgery right away if possible, or following preoperative neoadjuvant therapy if suitable. Early-stage invasive lobular carcinoma can be treated similarly to invasive ductal carcinoma with surgical excision and radiation therapy.

Given the high percentage of cases that test positive for ER and PR, adjuvant hormone therapy is recommended. Chemotherapy has minimal benefits for individuals with invasive lobular carcinoma due to low proliferation rates in most cases. Age, lymph node status, tumor size, Ki-67 biomarker, and hormonal state can all be connected with both recurrence and survival, and hence histology cannot be considered the main predictor [1, 2, 5, 9–11, 13, 15, 18–20, 27, 28, 31–46].

3.6 Lobular Carcinoma In Situ

3.6.1 Introduction

LCIS is both a risk factor and a nonessential precursor to breast malignancy. Following a diagnosis of classic LCIS, the relative risk of invasive cancer is roughly 9–10 times higher than in the general population. LCIS and ILC have similar copy number changes and somatic mutations. A subgroup of LCIS is clonally linked to synchronous or subsequent invasive breast cancer. Classic LCIS diagnosed via core biopsy with concordant imaging and pathologic findings does not require surgical excision. The margin status of classical LCIS is not mentioned. Active monitoring and chemoprevention are two treatment options for classic LCIS. The presence of variant LCIS in a needle core biopsy specimen necessitates surgical removal, regardless of radiologic-pathologic concordance [1, 2, 18, 39].

In 1941, Foote and Stewart identified LCIS as a rare breast cancer that originates in lobules and terminal ducts [1]. They recorded all of the main morphologic aspects of LCIS, which are still true and accurate today. (1) LCIS is a microscopic discovery, not a clinical diagnostic. It cannot be recognized overtly. (2) LCIS has distinct morphological characteristics: "The cells lose polarity, varying in shape while remaining surprisingly uniform in size." (3) LCIS is multifocal: "it is always a disease of multiple foci" [1, 2, 18, 39].

The aforementioned qualities define the so-called classic form of LCIS. Although classic LCIS is a risk factor and non-obligate precursor of invasive breast cancer, it is currently treated as a benign lesion that does not require complete removal or margin inspection. For patients with classic LCIS, hormonal chemoprevention is suggested. The American Joint Committee on Cancer (AJCC)2's eighth edition of TNM staging no longer stages LCIS as Tis3.

Classic LCIS (LCIS) is typically discovered as an accidental discovery in a breast needle core biopsy or surgical excision material intended to treat another lesion. It is so impossible to estimate the true incidence of LCIS. LCIS is detected in 0.5–1.5% of benign breast biopsies and 1.8–2.5% of all breast biopsies [4–7]. A population-based analysis using data from the Surveillance, Epidemiology, and End Results (SEER) program found that the incidence of LCIS in women without prior history of in situ or invasive breast cancer increased from 0.90/100,000 person year in 1978–1980 to 3.19/100,000 person year in 1996–1998.8, 9. The increased use of mammographic screening and biopsy of mammographically indeterminate or worrisome lesions are most likely to blame for the rise in LCIS cases [1, 2, 18, 39].

3.6.2 Pathophysiology and Histopathology

LCIS is a proliferation centered in the terminal ductal-lobular units (TDLUs) made up of neoplastic cells that fill and expand the majority (>50%) of the acini. It is also usual to see pagetoid extension into the terminal ducts, as well as LCIS cell proliferation beneath the ductal epithelium [1, 2, 18, 39]. Classic LCIS is characterized by monomorphic, dyshesive proliferation of non-polarized cells with round to oval shapes, and inconspicuous cytoplasm. The cells' nuclei are tiny, round to oval, with a smooth nuclear membrane and inconspicuous nucleoli. The cell borders are unclear. Intracytoplasmic vacuoles are prevalent, and signet-ring cells can develop. Mitotic activity is not present (see Fig. 3.18) [1, 2, 18, 39].

Classic LCIS cells might have minimal cytoplasm ("small cells" or "type A" cells) or be significantly larger ("large cell" or "type B"), with slightly more plentiful cytoplasm, bigger nuclei, and more conspicuous nucleoli. The two cell types can coexist in the same patient, breast, or lobule. In the absence of necrosis or

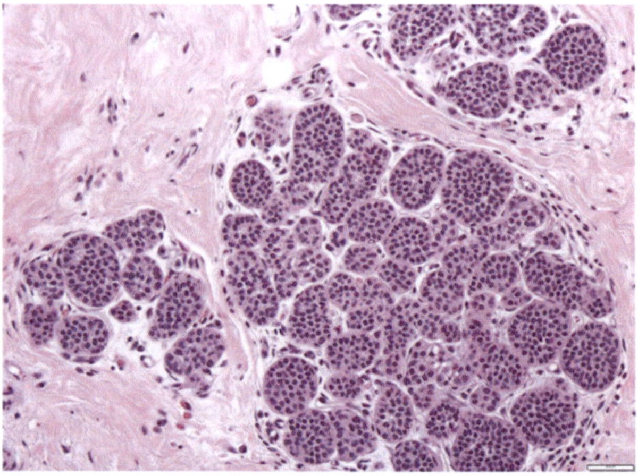

Fig. 3.18 Histopathology of LCIS
The acini are expanded by monomorphic, evenly spaced dyshesive cells with low-grade nuclear atypia. Magnification 200× [1, 2, 18, 39]

significant nuclear pleomorphism, LCIS constituted primarily of big cells is classed as traditional LCIS [1, 2, 18, 39].

The phrase "lobular neoplasia" refers to a variety of lesions, including atypical lobular hyperplasia (ALH) and classic LCIS. ALH cells are morphologically similar to those of typical LCIS, but proliferation is limited to fewer than 50% of the acini of the terminal duct lobular units, and none are significantly enlarged. ALH has identical genetic changes and immunohistochemistry profiles to conventional LCIS, and the two lesions frequently coexist. ALH is related to a 4-to-five-fold increase in the chance of developing breast cancer (see Figs. 3.19 and 3.20) [1, 2, 18, 39].

3.6.2.1 LCIS Variants: Pleomorphic LCIS (P-LCIS)

The word "pleomorphic" was first used to describe a type of invasive lobular carcinoma (ILC) that has the same infiltrative pattern as classic ILC (single-cell files or targetoid arrangement of dyshesive cells) but has significant nuclear pleomorphism. Pleomorphic ILC (P-ILC) is distinguished from traditional ILC by larger cells with round to oval shapes, copious cytoplasm, and large hyperchromatic nuclei that are slightly off-center and have conspicuous nucleoli. Binucleation is prevalent. The cytoplasm is typically eosinophilic and somewhat grainy or frothy. Intracytoplasmic vacuoles resembling those found in classic ILC are prevalent. Mitotic activity is observed. Some P-ILCs exhibit apocrine differentiation [1, 2, 18, 39].

3.6.2.2 LCIS Variants: LCIS with Necrosis (Also Known as "florid" LCIS)

LCIS with necrosis is a proliferative lesion that has the cytologic features of classic LCIS, such as cell dyshesion and type A or type B morphology, but is distinguished by massive expansion of the acini (at least 50 cells across the diameter of an acinus) and central necrosis, which preclude the diagnosis of classic LCIS (see Table 3.1). Calcifications are commonly found in necrotic foci [1, 2, 18, 39]. This lesion is also known as the "florid" LCIS. LCIS with necrosis typically occurs at a later age than

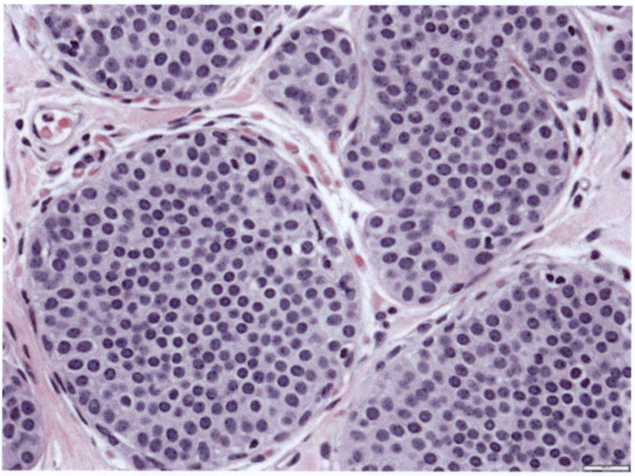

Fig. 3.19 Classic LCIS type A cells [1, 2, 18, 39]

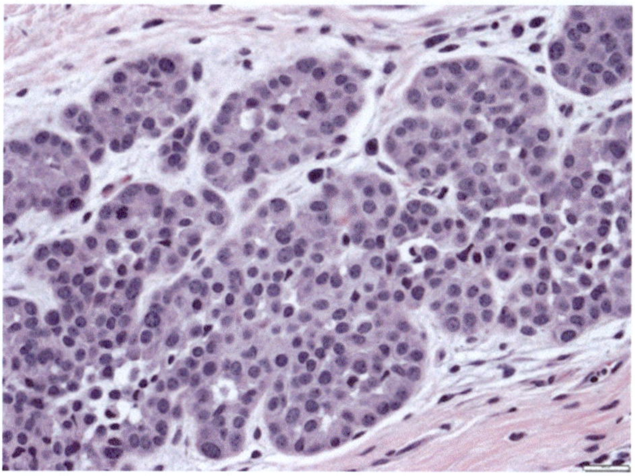

Fig. 3.20 Classic LCIS type B cells [1, 2, 18, 39]

Table 3.1 Variants of LCIS subtypes [1, 2, 18, 39]

	Classic LCIS	Pleomorphic LCIS	Florid LCIS
Relationship to menopause	Pre-	Post-	Post-
Mean age of diagnosis	50	60	60
Comedo necrosis	No	Can be present	Can be present
Calcification	Rare	Can be present	Can be present
Pleomorphism	Minimal	Marked (>4× lymphocyte)	Mild
B-code	B3	B5a	B4
Risk of upgrade on biopsy	1–4%[a]	33% (18–65%)	27% (17–45%)

[a]https://www.sciencedirect.com/science/article/abs/pii/S1756231722001906

standard LCIS and is frequently associated with aggressive cancer. Fadare et al. described 18 cases of LCIS with comedo type necrosis, 12 (67%) of which had concomitant invasive cancer, the most common being ILC with classic morphology. Like P-LCIS, LCIS with necrosis closely resembles solid DCIS [1, 2, 18, 39].

Immunohistochemistry reveals that normal mammary glands, DCIS, and the majority of invasive ductal carcinomas (IDCs) have strong and continuous E-cadherin membrane staining. In contrast, ILC and LCIS, including all LCIS variations, are distinguished by the absence or abnormal expression of the E-cadherin protein. An immunohistochemical stain for E-cadherin is commonly used to identify lobular from ductal lesions, and it is notably beneficial in distinguishing LCIS variations from DCIS in instances with equivocal shape. The majority of LCIS cases show total loss of E-cadherin staining; however in other cases, E-cadherin expression is reduced, with dispersed cells showing dot-like discontinuous and weak membranous staining or patchy cytoplasmic staining [1, 2, 18, 39].

3.6.3 Clinical Evaluation and Imaging

LCIS occurs mostly in premenopausal women, with a mean and median age at diagnosis of 49 and 50 years, respectively (range 20–80s). LCIS is multicentric in 60–80% of cases, and bilateral in 20–60%. Recent investigations suggest that classical LCIS may be associated with clustered amorphous or granular mammographic calcifications, or heterogeneous nonmass-like enhancement with persistent enhancement kinetics on MRI [13, 17]. LCIS variants, such as pleomorphic LCIS and LCIS with central necrosis, are frequently diagnosed mammographically due to concomitant pleomorphic calcifications. They can also present as a mass lesion with or without associated calcification [1, 2, 18, 39] (Fig. 2.21).

LCIS is frequently missed by mammography and discovered as an incidental finding on standard screening mammograms, mainly due to microcalcifications (see Fig. 3.22). LCIS, a high-risk lesion, can mimic aggressive cancer on ultrasound (see Fig. 3.23) [1, 2, 18, 39].

3.6.4 Treatment and Management

Historically, mastectomy was suggested for women with LCIS due to the higher chance of developing invasive breast cancer. Haagensen et al. pioneered the concept that "when it (LCIS) occurs alone without accompanying infiltrating carcinoma [47], it is a distinctive benign disease which predisposes to subsequent carcinoma" and urged a more conservative strategy of close follow-up as an alternative to mastectomy (refer to Fig. 3.21). LCIS is widely recognized as a risk factor and non-obligate precursor to breast cancer. Observation alone is the ideal management method. Chemoprevention counseling with tamoxifen or aromatase inhibitors is advised.

The National Comprehensive Cancer Network (NCCN) guidelines indicate that patients be followed up with physical examinations every 6–12 months [29], as well as annual diagnostic mammograms. In the eighth edition of the American Joint Committee on Cancer (AJCC) staging system, LCIS is no longer classified as pathologic tumor in situ (pTis) category 3. Randomized controlled clinical trials

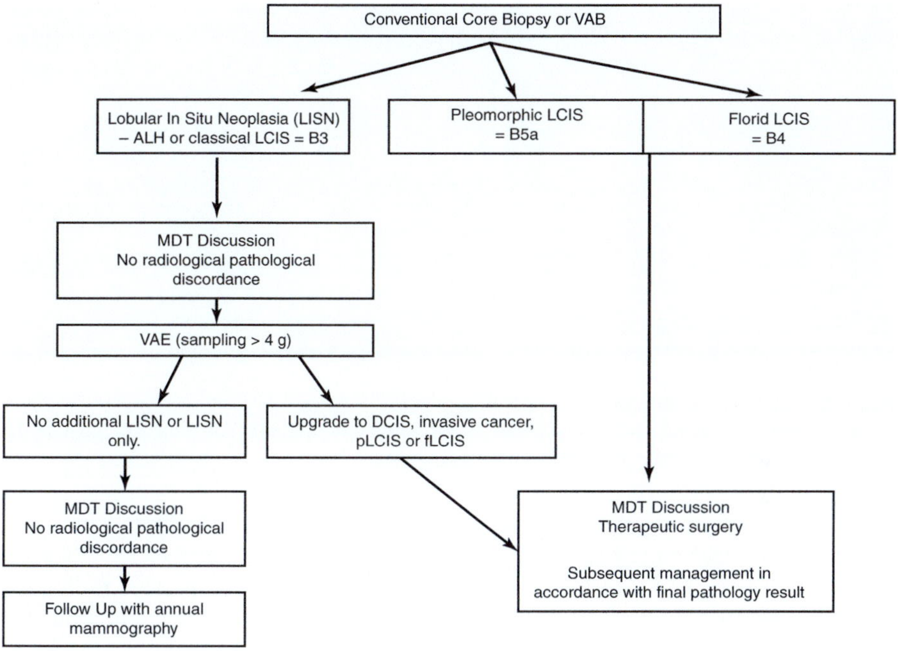

Fig. 3.21 Biopsy pathway related to LCIS findings [1, 2, 18, 39]

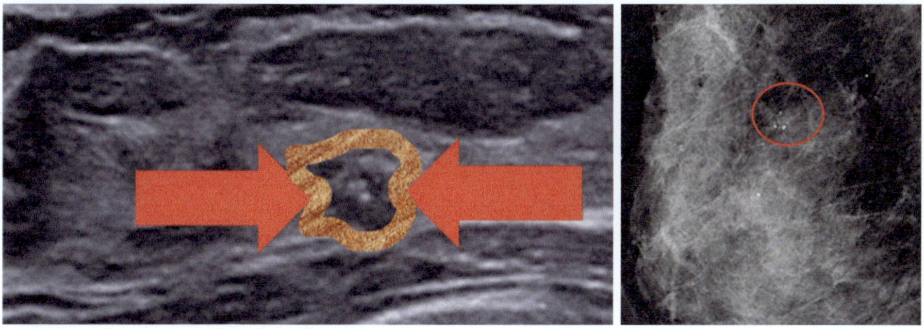

Fig. 3.22 LCIS on mammography

support the use of tamoxifen or aromatase inhibitors for risk reduction in women at high risk of breast cancer [1, 2, 18, 39].

P-LCIS is rare without concurrent invasive cancer, and hence descriptions of its natural history are anecdotal. There are no randomized prospective clinical study data available. There is currently no consensus on treatment recommendations for P-LCIS [1, 2, 18, 39].

The World Health Organization's 2012 consensus classification states that "in the absence of better information on the natural history of pleomorphic LCIS, caution should be exercised in recommending more aggressive management strategies,

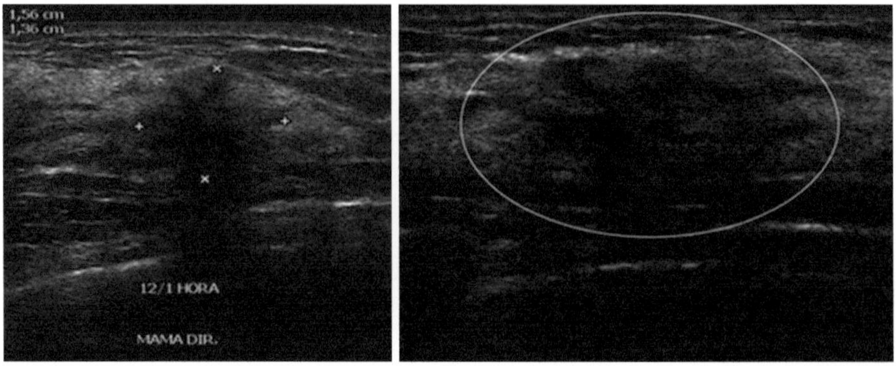

Fig. 3.23 LCIS on ultrasound
Ultrasonography showing a hypoechoic noduliform formation, irregular and poorly defined, in the palpation region in the upper quadrants of the right breast

such as excision to negative margins or mastectomy as a routine practice after a diagnostic surgical biopsy reveals pleomorphic LCIS." According to NCCN standards, some types of LCIS (pleomorphic LCIS) may have comparable biological activity to DCIS. Clinicians may consider total excision with negative margins for pleomorphic LCIS, although this may result in a high mastectomy rate with no demonstrated therapeutic benefit. There is no evidence to justify utilizing radiation in this scenario [1, 2, 18, 39, 42, 48, 49].

3.7 Metastases

3.7.1 Introduction

Metastatic breast cancer, also known as stage IV breast cancer, is when breast cancer has progressed to another part of the body, typically the bones, lungs, brain, or liver.

Metastasis refers to the process by which cancer spreads. Metastasis occurs when cancer cells break out from the primary tumor in the breast and spread to other regions of the body. Cancer cells spread through the bloodstream or lymphatic system, which eliminates germs, viruses, and cell waste [42, 48, 49].

Breast cancer can return in another place of the body months or years after being diagnosed and treated. This is known as metastatic or distant recurrence. Almost 30% of women with early-stage breast cancer develop metastatic disease [118, 119].

Key Facts of Metastatic Breast Cancer

- Rare, < 1% of breast malignancies.
- Can be initially misdiagnosed due to nonspecific/overlapping clinical, radiologic, morphologic and immunophenotypic features with primary breast carcinoma, especially if inadequate clinical history is provided.
- Accurate identification of extramammary metastases is critical to avoid unnecessary surgery and inappropriate treatment.
- Metastases to the breast represent 0.2–1.3% of breast malignancies.
- More common in women.
- Median age in fifth decade but can occur in pediatric patients.

3.7.2 Pathophysiology and Histopathology

Lymphoma, melanoma, sarcoma (uterine leiomyosarcoma, rhabdomyosarcoma, liposarcoma), and carcinoma (frequent primary sites include gynecologic, lung, gastrointestinal, genitourinary, head, and neck) can all metastasis to the breast [42, 48, 49].

The most common main sites are cutaneous malignant melanoma, lung, and ovary.

The most prevalent primary tumors in pediatric children are lymphoma and rhabdomyosarcoma.

Breast lymphoma can be caused by either primary or secondary systemic involvement [42, 48, 49].

Metastasis is the final stage in the progression of cancer and is usually fatal. Cutaneous metastases (CMs) represent 2% of all skin cancers. Breast cancer accounts for over 70% of all CMs in women. Because CM is typically linked with a poor prognosis, developing treatment methods for these individuals remains a significant therapeutic issue. Identifying molecular markers in primary breast cancer that predict CMs, as well as determining the molecular distinctions between main tumors and metastases, is critical for developing new therapeutic methods [42, 48, 49].

3.7.3 Clinical Evaluation and Imaging

Clinical signs of breast cancer metastases can manifest in various ways throughout the body, indicating the spread of cancer to other organs and tissues. Persistent back, bone, or joint pain may occur, often resisting relief through typical measures. Neurological symptoms, such as numbness, weakness, or difficulty urinating—either through incontinence or the inability to urinate—may arise, suggesting nerve compression in the spine. Respiratory symptoms, including a constant dry cough, shortness of breath, and chest pain, can signal lung involvement, while gastrointestinal symptoms like loss of appetite, abdominal bloating, pain, or tenderness might indicate metastasis to the digestive organs. Persistent nausea, vomiting, or unexplained weight loss may also develop, along with jaundice, a yellowing of the skin and eyes, suggesting liver involvement. Neurological signs may include severe headaches, vision problems like blurry or double vision, seizures, loss of balance, confusion, and persistent fatigue, highlighting potential brain involvement. These symptoms collectively emphasize the importance of timely assessment and management for patients with metastatic breast cancer [42, 48, 49].

Key Facts Regarding Clinical Signs of Metastatic Breast Cancer

- The majority of patients have a history of malignancy, typically with previous or concurrent metastases to other non-mammary locations.
- In 11–30% of instances, breast metastasis is the initial manifestation of an undetected extramammary cancer.
- Melanoma and ovarian cancer can show a long delay between initial malignancy and breast metastasis.
- Frequently manifests as a single, rapidly developing, tangible mass.
- Can occur with axillary lymphadenopathy.
- Presentation can resemble inflammatory breast cancer.

In diagnosing a breast lesion, the possibility of a non-mammary metastasis should be considered, especially when clinical, radiologic, or histomorphologic features appear atypical. A thorough clinical history is essential to arrive at an accurate diagnosis, as patients often have a known history of advanced, non-breast malignancy. When clinical evaluation and imaging do not clearly distinguish between primary breast cancer and metastasis, a biopsy is typically performed. The presence of a definitive in situ component in the biopsy can help rule out metastasis, confirming a primary breast origin [42, 48, 49]. However, the absence of an in situ component does not entirely exclude the possibility of a non-mammary metastasis, as not all primary mammary carcinomas exhibit an in situ component. In most cases, an immunohistochemical workup is necessary for diagnostic confirmation [42, 48, 49].

From a radiologic perspective, imaging features of non-mammary metastases in the breast can vary based on the origin and location of the primary tumor. Typically, these metastases appear as well-defined, discrete, rounded masses with less spiculation than primary breast cancers. Often, they initially present as unilateral, solitary masses; however, with disease progression, they may appear as multiple or bilateral masses. Calcifications are generally uncommon, except in cases of serous carcinoma originating from the ovary [42, 48, 49].

To assess for metastatic disease in breast cancer, a complete blood count (CBC) and liver function tests are commonly performed [42, 48, 49]. An oncologist may also decide to measure specific tumor markers, such as serum carcinoembryonic antigen (CEA), cancer antigen (CA) 15–3, or CA 27–29, and may recommend bone scanning based on individual patient factors. Indications for bone scanning typically include the presence of bone pain, elevated serum alkaline phosphatase, or a diagnosis of stage III or IV cancer. In cases where abdominal metastasis is suspected, an abdominal CT scan is advised if there are abnormal liver test results, findings from an abdominal or pelvic examination, or a diagnosis of stage III or IV cancer. A chest CT may be performed for patients experiencing pulmonary symptoms, like shortness of breath, or if the cancer has reached stage III or IV. Additionally, MRI is frequently used by surgeons in preoperative planning due to its accuracy in determining tumor size, involvement of the chest wall, and the number of tumors present [42, 48, 49].

3.7.4 Treatment and Management

Although systemic medications are the primary treatment for stage IV breast cancer, surgery, radiation therapy, and localized chemotherapy are also employed. These can help treat breast cancer in a specific area of the body, but they are unlikely to eliminate the cancer entirely. These treatments are more likely to be used to prevent or treat cancer-related symptoms or consequences [21, 22, 42, 48–50].

Radiation therapy and/or surgery may also be employed in specific cases, such as:

- When the breast tumor creates an open or painful incision in the breast (or chest).
- To treat a small number of metastases in a specific region, such as the brain.
- To prevent or cure bone fractures.
- When a malignancy presses against the spinal cord.
- To treat a blocked blood artery in the liver.
- To alleviate pain or other symptoms throughout the body.

3.8 Lymphoma

3.8.1 Introduction

Lymphoma is a very rare breast neoplasm. It could be primary or secondary, depending on whether there is lymphoma elsewhere in the body. Breast lymphoma is most commonly diagnosed as a painless palpable mass that is indistinguishable from breast cancer, despite the fact that treatment regimens for these two neoplasms differ greatly. Knowledge of the various mammographic and sonographic appearances of breast lymphoma should lead to more frequent detection of this uncommon malignancy. Proper identification of this neoplasm is critical for appropriate treatment planning and avoiding needless and potentially hazardous surgery [21, 22, 42, 48–50].

3.8.2 Pathophysiology and Histopathology

Wiseman and Liao originally defined primary breast lymphoma in 1972 [21, 22, 42, 48–50]. The following diagnostic criteria were proposed: breast as the location of presentation, breast tissue in close proximity to lymphomatous infiltration, lack of disseminated disease beyond the ipsilateral axillary lymph nodes, and no prior lymphoma diagnosis. This definition has remained unchanged until today. However, it only includes stage I (breast-limited) and stage II (limited to the breast and ipsilateral axillary ganglia) tumors. Its pathogenesis is uncertain; however, it is thought to originate from mucosa-associated lymphoid tissue (MALT), lymphoid tissue near breast ducts and lobes, or even intramammary lymph nodes [21, 22, 42, 48–50].

The most common histological type is diffuse large B-cell lymphoma, but up to 44% of patients may have MALT lymphomas. Other less common variations include Burkitt's lymphoma, marginal zone lymphoma, small-cell lymphocytic lymphoma, and large-cell anaplastic lymphoma [21, 22, 42, 48–50].

3.8.3 Clinical Evaluation and Imaging

A few identifying traits may be useful in determining the difference between primary and secondary breast lymphoma, albeit they are not pathognomonic in themselves. Secondary breast lymphoma tumors, unlike primary illness, frequently have smaller dimensions when they first appear. Previous studies [21, 22] reported that the average diameter of a tumor in secondary breast lymphoma was 2.8 cm, compared to 4.6 cm in primary breast lymphoma.

This conclusion could be explained in part by the fact that the duration of symptoms prior to clinical and radiologic testing may be shorter in individuals with known lymphomatous illness. Similarly, the number of intramammary masses has been found to be larger in secondary than primary breast lymphoma, consistent with the total amount of primary vs. secondary lymphomatous disease. Parenchymal breast involvement combined with bilateral axillary lymph node enlargement may indicate lymphoma, particularly secondary breast lymphoma, while extensive metastatic breast cancer may also show similarly [21, 22, 42, 48–50].

The most common mammographic finding is intramammary masses, which are typically round or oval in form with constricted or slightly lobulated edges (see Figs. 3.24, 3.25, and 3.26). Calcific deposits and spiculated edges are absent, and architectural distortion is uncommon. High-grade lymphomas are more likely to cause diffuse breast enlargement, whereas low- to intermediate-grade neoplasms show a more nodular appearance [21, 22, 42, 48–50].

Breast lymphoma presents sonographically as a hypoechoic to nearly anechoic round or oval-shaped mass with well-defined edges, with or without posterior acoustic enhancement. Although few studies have detailed the magnetic resonance imaging (MRI) characteristics of breast lymphoma, significant aspects have been identified thus far. On T2-weighted images, lesions are often hyperintense in

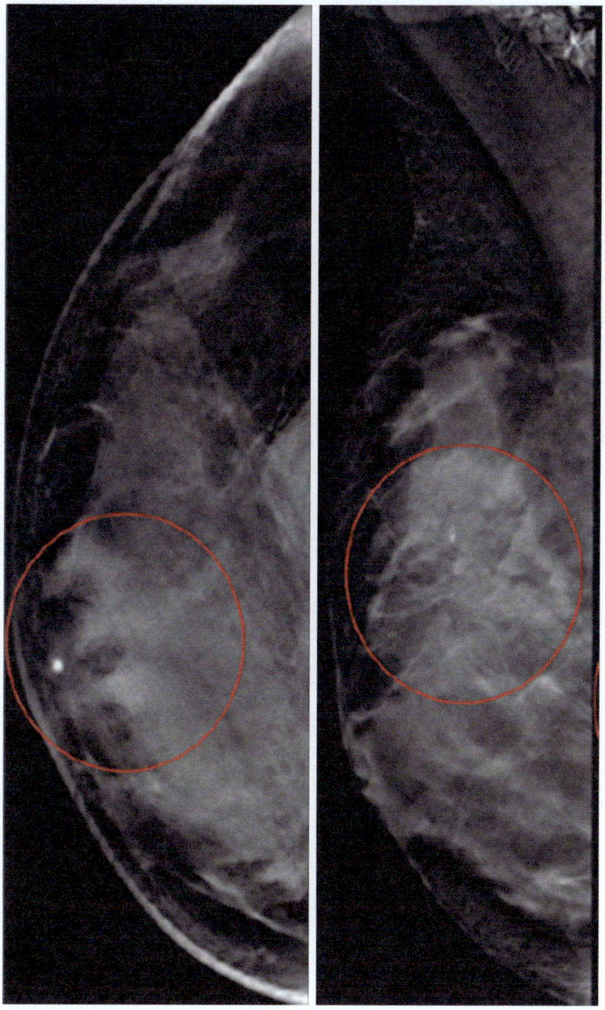

Fig. 3.24 Dense breast parenchyma with T-cell breast lymphoma [24]

comparison to the surrounding breast parenchyma, while T1-weighted images are isointense [21, 22, 42, 48–50].

3.8.4 Treatment and Management

The treatment of breast lymphoma is still somewhat contentious; nonetheless, specific criteria have been established. Patients who underwent mastectomy, either alone or in combination with treatment, perished from lymphoma. It has been suggested that this was caused by a delay in receiving proper systemic treatment. Correct diagnosis through tissue sampling is therefore critical to avoid the morbidity and mortality associated with unneeded surgery. Alternatively, numerous studies

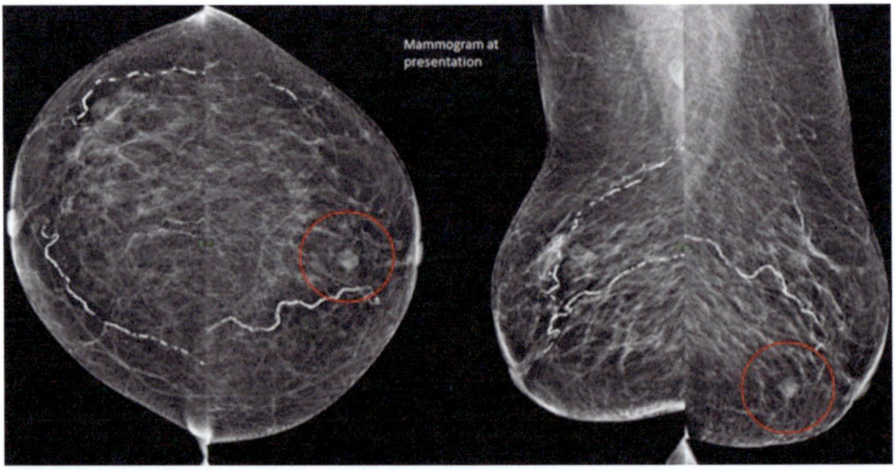

Fig. 3.25 CC and MLO view demonstrating lymphoma. Note the bilateral benign vascular calcifications [24]

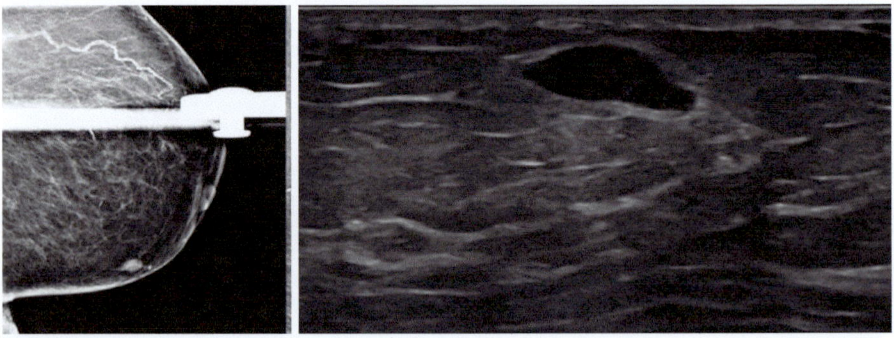

Fig. 3.26 Additional imaging of the breast indicating lymphoma [24]

have proposed a treatment strategy based on combination chemotherapy with or without concurrent radiation [21, 22, 42, 48–50].

3.9 Inflammatory Breast Cancer

3.9.1 Introduction

Inflammatory breast cancer is a rare and highly aggressive illness in which cancer cells obstruct lymph arteries in the breast surface. This kind of breast cancer is known as "inflammatory" because the breast appears swollen, red, or inflamed. Inflammatory breast cancer is uncommon, accounting for 1–5% of all breast cancers diagnosed in the United States. Most inflammatory breast cancers are invasive ductal carcinomas, which means they started in the milk ducts of the breast and spread beyond them [25, 51–53].

Inflammatory breast cancer spreads swiftly, frequently within weeks or months. Inflammatory breast cancer is classified as stage III or IV, based on whether it has migrated to surrounding lymph nodes or other organs [25, 51–53].

Additional Features of Inflammatory Breast Cancer

- Compared with other types of breast cancer, inflammatory breast cancer tends to be diagnosed at younger ages.
- Inflammatory breast cancer is more common and diagnosed at younger ages in African American women than in White women.
- Inflammatory breast tumors are frequently hormone receptor negative, which means they cannot be treated with hormone therapies, such as tamoxifen, that interfere with the growth of cancer cells fueled by estrogen.
- Inflammatory breast cancer is more common in obese women than in women of normal weight [25, 51–53].

Inflammatory breast cancer, like other kinds of breast cancer, can affect males, but typically at a later age than in women. The prognosis for a cancer patient is frequently defined as the likelihood that the malignancy will be successfully treated and the patient will recover entirely. A cancer patient's prognosis is influenced by various factors such as cancer kind and location, stage, age, general health, and therapy response. Because inflammatory breast cancer usually grows fast and aggressively spreads to other parts of the body, women diagnosed with this disease do not live as long as women diagnosed with other types of breast cancer [25, 51–53].

3.9.2 Pathophysiology and Histopathology

The American Joint Committee on Cancer (AJCC) tumor-node-metastasis (TNM) staging system for breast cancer classifies IBC as an uncommon subtype of locally advanced breast cancer (T4d). The most common histotypes in noninflammatory BC (n-IBC) are invasive ductal carcinoma (IDC) and invasive lobular carcinoma (ILC), both of which have distinct clinic-pathological and molecular profiles, prognoses, and treatment responses [25, 51–53].

IBC's clinical characteristics are well documented, and however its histology is not. In fact, no histological differentiation between lobular and ductal subtypes has been described in IBC [25, 51–53]. Thus, it is unclear if it reflects a heterogeneous group, such as n-IBC, or a totally homogenous unit.

IBC is distinguished by the presence of many dermal tumor emboli in the papillary and reticular dermis of the skin that covers the breast. In patients with IBC, emboli are often more numerous and larger than in non-IBCs. Embolic cells are often high in nuclear grade and have a ductal character. The majority of tumor emboli-filled areas in the dermis lack red blood cells and are thus classified as lymphatic.

The shape of cells in the skin of IBC patients is exceedingly diverse. Areas within and outside of the zone of erythema and edema may appear histologically identical, with lymphatic tumor emboli present. The presence of lymphovascular tumor emboli in the dermis helps with the clinical diagnosis of IBC. However, their absence cannot rule out an IBC [25, 51–53].

3.9.3 Clinical Evaluation and Imaging

Symptoms of inflammatory breast cancer include swelling (edema) and redness (erythema) in one-third or more of the breast (see Fig. 3.27). The skin of the breast may also seem pink, reddish purple, or bruised. Additionally, the skin may have ridges or appear pitted, similar to orange skin (known as "peau d'orange"). The symptoms are produced by an accumulation of fluid (lymph) in the breast skin. This fluid buildup happens when cancer cells block lymph veins in the skin, blocking normal lymph passage through the tissue. A solid tumor in the breast can occasionally be felt during a physical exam, but most of the time it cannot [25, 51–53].

The abnormal mammography findings in this setting have been extensively discussed in the literature, with thickening of the skin being the most common, occurring in 84% of cases in Günhan-Bilgen's study [25, 51–53]. This thickening, which is typically more noticeable in areas with low breast volume, appears to begin in the inferior areolar region before swiftly spreading across the skin covering. As with most imaging phenomena, it appears to be associated with tumoral obstruction of the lymphatics, resulting in impaired drainage, particularly of the skin. The second most prevalent symptom is trabecular thickening, which occurs in 81% of patients and is histologically similar to skin thickening [25, 51–53].

Furthermore, intramammary edema typically causes an overall rise in breast density, which has a negative impact on mammography reading, particularly when searching for subjacent tumors. In contrast to Dershaw's 1994 study,

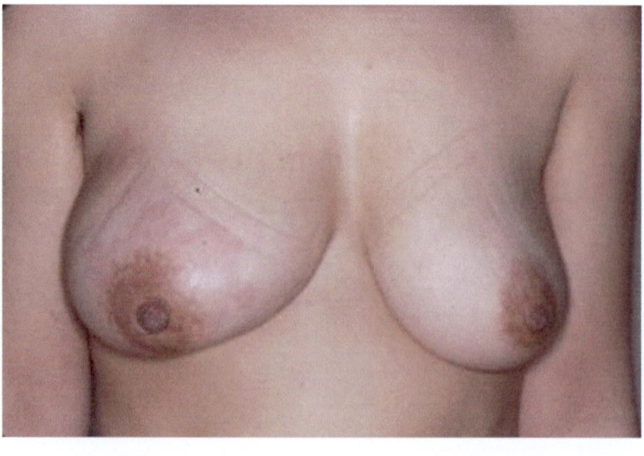

Fig. 3.27 Clinical appearance of IBC
Image represents inflammatory breast cancer associating periareolar erythema with skin thickening, an increase in breast volume and nipple retraction [25]

Günhan-Bilgen discovered an intramammary mass in only 16% of instances, with the majority of lesions being focal asymmetric density (61%). Architectural abnormalities are infrequent, and the overall increase in breast density occurs in only 37% of cases [25, 51–53].

Microcalcifications are present in around 56% of cases, distinguishing this condition from locally progressed malignancy, which is significantly more commonly associated with lesions of widespread intraductal carcinoma. The literature contains a wide variation in terms of the percentage of masses and microcalcifications identified in this inflammatory context, with some older studies failing to distinguish between primary inflammatory cancer and secondary inflammation of advanced cancer, which is much more likely to present with a mass and associated microcalcifications [25, 51–53].

Inflammatory cancer microcalcifications can arise in a variety of ways (see Fig. 3.28), with benign microcalcifications distributed widely in approximately 10% of cases. Nonetheless, when they appear, they are typically ACR 4 or even 5. The mammography shows nipple retraction in 43% of instances, which is consistent with clinical findings. Finally, in 24% of cases, mammography reveals axillary adenomegaly (see Figs. 3.29, 3.30, and 3.31) [25, 51–53].

Minimum Criteria for a Diagnosis of Inflammatory Breast Cancer Include the Following

- A rapid onset of erythema (redness), edema (swelling), and a peau d'orange appearance (ridged or pitted skin) and/or abnormal breast warmth, with or without a lump that can be felt.
- The above-mentioned symptoms have been present for less than 6 months.
- The erythema covers at least a third of the breast.
- Initial biopsy samples from the affected breast show invasive carcinoma.

3.9.4 Treatment and Management

Inflammatory breast cancer is typically treated initially with systemic chemotherapy to reduce tumor size, followed by surgery to remove the tumor, and then radiation therapy. This sequential treatment strategy is known as a multimodal approach. Research indicates that women with inflammatory breast cancer respond better to this multimodal approach, showing improved therapy responses and increased survival rates. The treatment modalities within this approach are varied and include several options [25, 51–53].

Neoadjuvant chemotherapy, administered before surgery, commonly involves anthracycline and taxane drugs. It is generally recommended that patients receive at least 6 cycles of this chemotherapy over 4–6 months before undergoing tumor removal, unless the disease shows continued progression, in which case surgery may proceed without delay. Targeted therapy is another option, especially as inflammatory breast cancers often overexpress the HER2 protein. Drugs like trastuzumab

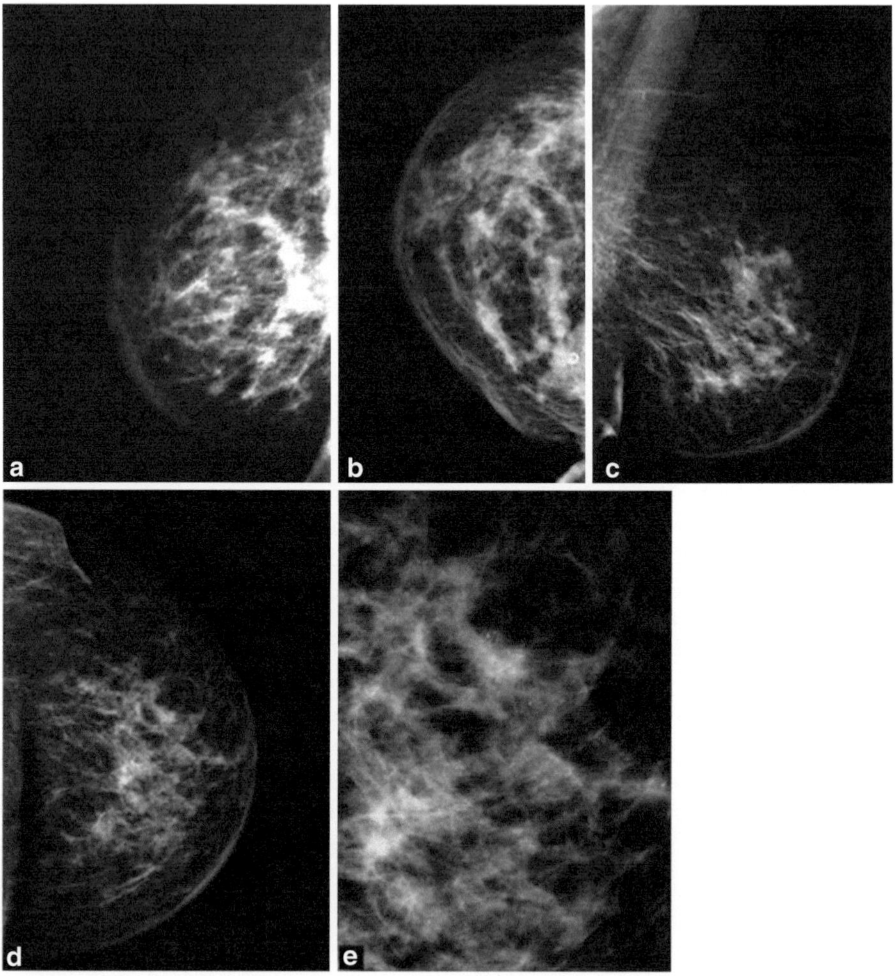

Fig. 3.28 Mammographic appearance of inflammatory breast cancer [25]. (**a** and **b**): MLO (**a**) and CC (**b**) incidence showing circumferential skin thickening, trabecular thickening, an overall increase in the density of the breast, and several images of poorly defined masses including a superior medial mass (with coil). Nipple retraction can also be seen; (**c**, **d**, and **e**): MLO (**c**), and CC (**d**) incidence and enlarged CC image (**e**) of another patient showing predominant periareolar skin thickening, with an overall increase in the density of the breast without a very clear mass. On the magnification view (**e**) diffuse pleomorphic microcalcifications can be seen

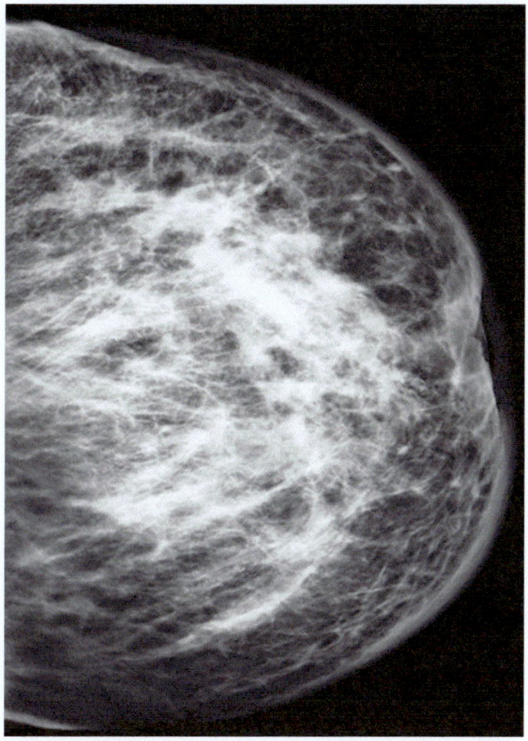

Fig. 3.29 Mammographic findings of inflammatory breast cancer [25, 51–53]

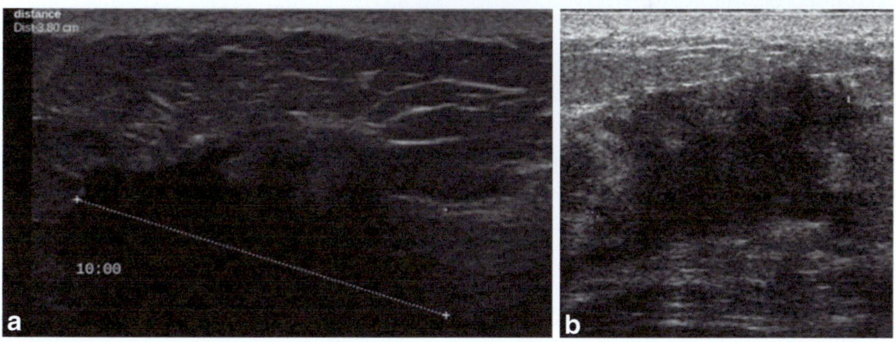

Fig. 3.30 Ultrasound image of inflammatory breast cancer
Image is seen with associated skin thickening and a hypoechoic shadowing mass [25, 51–53]

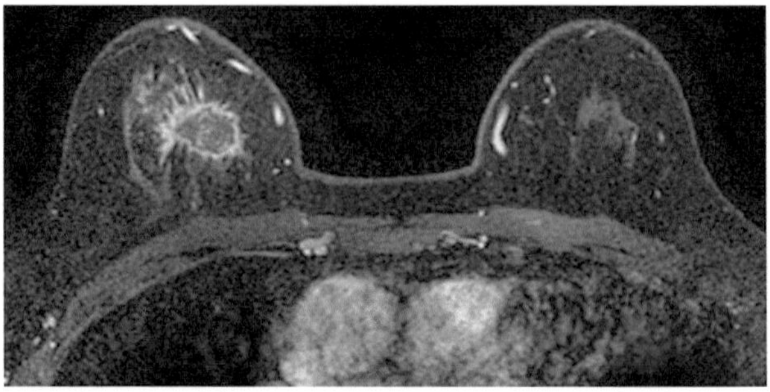

Fig. 3.31 MRI image of inflammatory breast cancer [54]

(Herceptin), which target HER2, may be used both in neoadjuvant and post-surgery (adjuvant) settings. Additionally, hormone therapy may be considered for cases where cancer cells have hormone receptors. Drugs such as tamoxifen and aromatase inhibitors like letrozole work by either blocking estrogen binding or inhibiting estrogen production, leading to the death of estrogen-dependent cancer cells [25, 51–53].

Surgery for inflammatory breast cancer typically involves a modified radical mastectomy, which entails removing the entire affected breast and most or all of the lymph nodes under the adjacent arm. The lining over the chest muscles is also often removed, although the chest muscles themselves are generally preserved, except in some cases where the smaller pectoralis minor muscle may also be removed. Following surgery, radiation therapy to the chest wall is a standard component of multimodal treatment. If the patient received trastuzumab before surgery, it may be continued during postoperative radiation therapy. Although breast reconstruction is possible for women with inflammatory breast cancer, experts often recommend delaying reconstruction until after radiation therapy to avoid interference with this critical treatment [25, 51–53].

Adjuvant therapy may be administered post-surgery to further reduce the risk of cancer recurrence. This therapy can include additional chemotherapy, hormone therapy, targeted therapy like trastuzumab, or a combination of these treatments to support long-term recovery and prevention [25, 51–53].

3.10 Phyllodes Tumor of Malignant Type

3.10.1 Introduction

Phyllodes tumors of the breast are rare fibroepithelial tumors with a wide variety of clinical characteristics. These tumors are classified as benign, borderline, or malignant depending on a variety of histopathological characteristics. The prognosis for phyllodes tumors is good, with local recurrence in around 15% of patients and distant recurrence in about 5–10%. The definitive primary treatment is a wide excision with a margin of more than 1 cm. Adjuvant systemic treatment has no established efficacy. Patients with locally recurrent disease should have a wide excision of the recurrence, with or without following radiation.

Consider all fibroadenomas to be possible phyllodes tumors unless proven otherwise, with a core biopsy conducted prior to surgery if the index of suspicion is elevated [55, 56].

3.10.2 Pathophysiology and Histopathology

Phyllodes tumors contain both epithelial and stromal elements, but the stroma is what distinguishes them histologically. These tumors have elongated ductal components and papillary protrusions of connective tissue lined with epithelium, which give them a leaf-like appearance. Marked stromal overgrowth and hypercellularity distinguish these lesions from more frequent fibroadenomas. These lesions are classified as benign, borderline, or malignant based on histologic criteria such as stromal cellular atypia, mitotic activity, stromal overgrowth, tumor margin type (circumscribed vs. infiltrative), and tumor necrosis. The reported incidence of each subtype varies greatly in the literature. In most major series, more than half are classified as benign, with just about 25% classified as cancer [55, 56].

The epithelial component of phyllodes tumors expresses estrogen and progesterone receptors, whereas the stromal component does not. In one series, 58% of the cells expressed epithelial estrogen receptors, while 75% expressed progesterone receptors. In this series, hormone receptor expression was associated to histologic grade, with estrogen and progesterone receptor expression found in 67% and 77% of benign, 43% and 84% of borderline, and 47% and 47% of malignant phyllodes tumors, respectively. All cancers had low levels of androgen receptors [55, 56].

The prevalence and significance of the tumor suppressor gene p53 in phyllodes tumors vary greatly among series. In some but not all series, p53 expression rises over the spectrum of benign to malignant phyllodes tumors. Clonal examination of phyllodes tumors reveals that the epithelial component is polyclonal, while the stromal component is monoclonal, indicating that the stroma is the neoplastic component of phyllodes tumors [55, 56].

3.10.3 Clinical Evaluation and Imaging

The most typical manifestation of a phyllodes tumor is a palpable breast mass that may be rapidly developing. These tumors can grow in two phases, and patients may seek medical attention only after seeing fast growth in a lesion that had previously been stable for years. Rarely, patients come with a mass discovered after routine screening mammography [55, 56]. Phyllodes tumors can grow to huge proportions; tumors larger than 20 cm have been documented in many series (see Figs. 3.32 and 3.33).

Many studies have found no link between tumor size and histologic subtype, owing to the fact that even benign phyllodes tumors can grow to be quite large [55, 56].

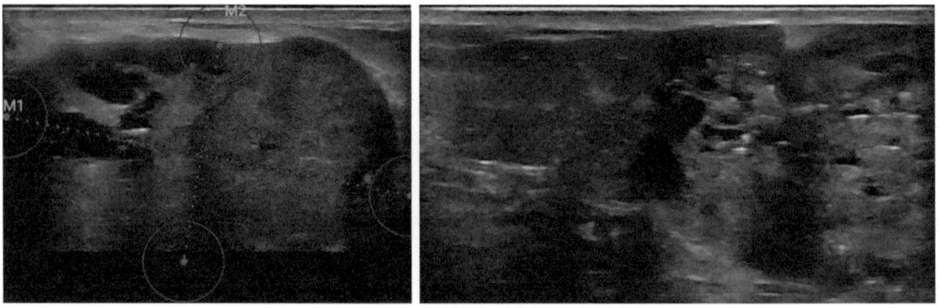

Fig. 3.32 Ultrasound appearance of malignant phyllodes tumor

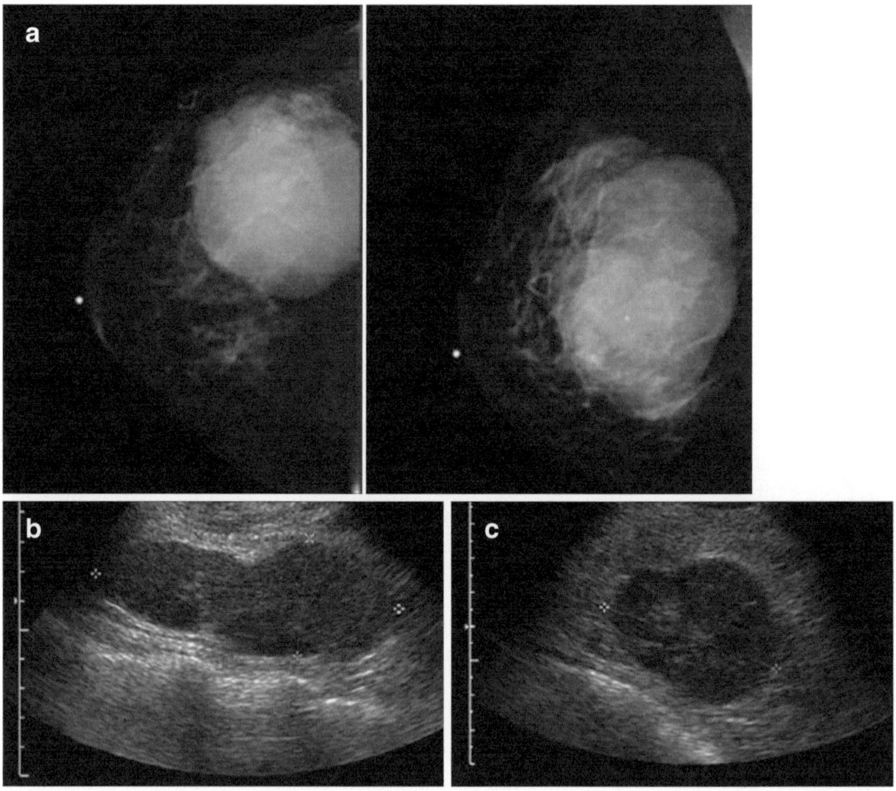

Fig. 3.33 Case images of a phyllodes tumor

On examination, the majority of patients have a smooth, round, well-defined, hard mass that is movable and painless. Large lesions may be associated with dilated veins visible on the skin, which can be stretched and attenuated. Nipple retraction, skin ulceration, chest wall invasion, and bloody nipple discharge have all been documented, and however these are extremely rare. Palpable axillary lymphadenopathy can be detected in up to 20% of patients, and however metastatic involvement of axillary lymph nodes is uncommon [55, 56].

The Paddington Clinicopathological Suspicion Score (see Table 3.2) was created to establish criteria for selecting individuals for core biopsy, which might be used in conjunction with current local practices. The goal of designing the score is to increase the rate of preoperative diagnosis [55, 56].

Phyllodes tumors appear at a median age of 45 years, but occurrences in teenagers and the elderly have been well documented. According to recent Surveillance, Epidemiology, and End Results (SEER) statistics, individuals with malignant phyllodes tumors have an average age at diagnosis of 50 years. Bilateral phyllodes tumors are uncommon, and one example of a phyllodes tumor developing in an accessory breast has been described. Furthermore, phyllodes tumors associated with gynecomastia have been recorded in men, as has a bilateral phyllodes tumor developing from an ectopic axillary breast tumor [55, 56].

On mammograms, phyllodes tumors appear as well-defined oval, round, or lobulated masses similar to fibroadenomas. The associated coarse microcalcifications are occasionally evident. Ultrasonography shows these lesions as solid, hypoechoic, well-defined masses. Ultrasound imaging shows a cystic region within a solid mass, indicating a phyllodes tumor (see Fig. 3.32).

Using fine needle aspiration (FNA) to diagnose a phyllodes tumor is associated with a high percentage of false negative outcomes and an overall accuracy of 63%. Because these tumors have such a diverse composition, poor sampling frequently jeopardizes FNA accuracy. Core biopsy, while having the same possibility for sample mistake, is associated with higher accuracy than FNA. In a recent article, Jacklin et al. determined that core biopsy may be the most helpful approach of preoperatively identifying phyllodes tumor [55, 56].

3.10.4 Treatment and Management

Local recurrence occurs in around 15% of individuals with phyllodes tumors, and it is more common after poor excision. Distant failure occurs in 5–10% of all instances, and in around 20% of malignant tumors. Metastatic potential appears to be determined by tumor biology, and local therapy appears to have no effect on this risk. Given these findings, the major surgical goal is to establish definitive local control [55, 56].

Table 3.2 The paddington clinicopathological suspicion score

Clinical findings	Sudden increase in size in longstanding breast lesion
	Apparent fibroadenoma >3 cm in diameter or in a patient >35 years
Imaging findings	Rounded borders/lobulated appearance at mammography
	Attenuation of cystic areas within a solid mass on ultrasound
Fine needle aspiration findings	Presence of hypercellular stromal fragments
	Indeterminate features
Any 2 features mandate core biopsy	

The preferred primary therapy is a wide local excision with margins of at least 1 cm. Microscopic tumor projections frequently extend into the pseudocapsule of normal compressed breast tissue that surrounds these lesions [55, 56].

To achieve a 1-cm microscopic margin, more tissue is usually removed than would be predicted based on gross inspection. Simple tumor enucleation, which is routinely employed in the treatment of fibroadenoma, is ineffective for phyllodes tumors [55, 56].

Historically, mastectomy was the primary surgical treatment for all phyllodes tumors. Breast-conservative techniques have recently gained popularity. In the Chaney et al. study, around half of the patients were treated with breast conservation and the other half with mastectomy. Only four local recurrences were detected, and they occurred similarly in both groups. Other large series have yielded similar results [55, 56].

However, given the low likelihood of local failure with breast-conserving surgery, breast conservation is the preferred primary therapy if negative margins can be attained while maintaining an acceptable cosmetic result. Total mastectomy is recommended when breast conservation is impossible due to the tumor's enormous size compared to the breast volume.

When phyllodes tumor is discovered after narrow margin excision, re-excision to obtain margins larger than 1 cm is recommended [55, 56].

3.11 Conclusion

This chapter included exploration of various types of breast cancer and malignant breast diseases, focusing on their diagnosis, histopathology, clinical imaging, and treatment. It begins with Atypical Breast Hyperplasia, discussing its histopathological characteristics and management strategies. Following this, the chapter delves into specific cancer types, including Ductal Carcinoma (both in situ and invasive forms) and Lobular Carcinoma, detailing each subtype's pathology, imaging techniques, and treatment options.

The chapter also examines less common breast malignancies like Metastatic Breast Disease, Lymphoma, Inflammatory Breast Cancer, emphasizing their unique clinical presentations and management.

Each section provides a structured analysis that includes the introduction to the disease type, insights into pathophysiology and histopathology, clinical imaging evaluations, and treatment protocols. The chapter concludes with a summary of the key points, enhancing the understanding of malignant breast disease management and providing comprehensive references for further reading.

References

1. Graziano L, Bitencourt AG, Guatelli CS, Souza JA, Osorio CA, Poli MR, et al. Lobular carcinoma in situ with atypical mass presentation: a case report. Rev Bras Ginecol Obstet. 2016;38(2):112–6.
2. Simpson PT, Gale T, Fulford LG, Reis-Filho JS, Lakhani SR. The diagnosis and management of pre-invasive breast disease: pathology of atypical lobular hyperplasia and lobular carcinoma in situ. Breast Cancer Res. 2003;5(5):258–62.

3. Bellini C, Nori Cucchiari J, Di Naro F, De Benedetto D, Bicchierai G, Franconeri A, et al. Breast lesions of uncertain malignant potential (B3) and the risk of breast cancer development: a long-term follow-up study. Cancers (Basel). 2023;15(13)
4. Fitzgibbons PL. Atypical lobular hyperplasia of the breast: a study of pathologists' responses in the college of American pathologists performance improvement program in surgical pathology. Arch Pathol Lab Med. 2000;124(3):463–4.
5. Malherbe K, Bresser P. Association between ultrasound morphologic features and histopathological findings of lobular carcinoma. J Med Radiat Sci. 2019;66(3):177–83.
6. Pathology of atypical lobular hyperplas
7. Nicosia L, Latronico A, Addante F, De Santis R, Bozzini AC, Montesano M, et al. Atypical ductal hyperplasia after vacuum-assisted breast biopsy: can we reduce the upgrade to breast cancer to an acceptable rate? Diagnostics (Basel). 2021;11(6)
8. Ehteshami Bejnordi B, Mullooly M, Pfeiffer RM, Fan S, Vacek PM, Weaver DL, et al. Using deep convolutional neural networks to identify and classify tumor-associated stroma in diagnostic breast biopsies. Mod Pathol. 2018;31(10):1502–12.
9. Evans N, Lyons K. The use of ultrasound in the diagnosis of invasive lobular carcinoma of the breast less than 10 mm in size. Clin Radiol. 2000;55(4):261–3.
10. Pointon KS, Cunningham DA. Ultrasound findings in pure invasive lobular carcinoma of the breast: comparison with matched cases of invasive ductal carcinoma of the breast. Breast. 1999;8(4):188–90.
11. Izumori A, Takebe K, Sato A. Ultrasound findings and histological features of ductal carcinoma in situ detected by ultrasound examination alone. Breast Cancer. 2010;17(2):136–41.
12. Orimo A, Gupta PB, Sgroi DC, Arenzana-Seisdedos F, Delaunay T, Naeem R, et al. Stromal fibroblasts present in invasive human breast carcinomas promote tumor growth and angiogenesis through elevated SDF-1/CXCL12 secretion. Cell. 2005;121(3):335–48.
13. Butler RS, Venta LA, Wiley EL, Ellis RL, Dempsey PJ, Rubin E. Sonographic evaluation of infiltrating lobular carcinoma. AJR Am J Roentgenol. 1999;172(2):325–30.
14. SM. Ductal carcinoma in situ. Publication Types. MeSH Terms PubMed Commons; 1992
15. Menezes GL, van den Bosch MA, Postma EL, El Sharouni MA, Verkooijen HM, van Diest PJ, et al. Invasive ductolobular carcinoma of the breast: spectrum of mammographic, ultrasound and magnetic resonance imaging findings correlated with proportion of the lobular component. Springerplus. 2013;2:621.
16. Thompson A, Brennan K, Cox A, Gee J, Harcourt D, Harris A, et al. Evaluation of the current knowledge limitations in breast cancer research: a gap analysis. Breast Cancer Res. 2008;10(2):R26.
17. Grimm LJ, Rahbar H, Abdelmalak M, Hall AH, Ryser MD. Ductal carcinoma in situ: state-of-the-art review. Radiology. 2022;302(2):246–55.
18. Chivukula M, Haynik DM, Brufsky A, Carter G, Dabbs DJ. Pleomorphic lobular carcinoma in situ (PLCIS) on breast core needle biopsies: clinical significance and immunoprofile. Am J Surg Pathol. 2008;32(11):1721–6.
19. Berg WA, Gilbreath PL. Multicentric and multifocal cancer: whole-breast US in preoperative evaluation. Radiology. 2000;214(1):59–66.
20. Berg WA, Gutierrez L, NessAiver MS, Carter WB, Bhargavan M, Lewis RS, et al. Diagnostic accuracy of mammography, clinical examination, US, and MR imaging in preoperative assessment of breast cancer. Radiology. 2004;233(3):830–49.
21. Moura C, Leite MI, Parreira R, Medeiros A. Primary breast lymphoma. J Surg Case Rep. 2020;2020(1):rjz405.
22. Kelli Y, Ha M, et al. Lymphoma in the breast. Radiology Report. 2013;26(2):146–8.
23. Jing H, Yang Y, Nishikawa RM. Regularization in retrieval-driven classification of clustered microcalcifications for breast cancer. Int J Biomed Imaging. 2012;2012:463408.
24. Tran MG, Cortes G, Choi HW, Young JJ, Tsai IS. Case-based review of breast lymphomas. Curr Radiol Rep. 2024;12(5):41–50.
25. Gunhan-Bilgen I, Ustun EE, Memis A. Inflammatory breast carcinoma: mammographic, ultrasonographic, clinical, and pathologic findings in 142 cases. Radiology. 2002;223(3):829–38.

26. Petroni S, Caldarola L, Scamarcio R, Giotta F, Latorre A, Mangia A, et al. FISH testing of HER2 immunohistochemistry 1+ invasive breast cancer with unfavorable characteristics. Oncol Lett. 2016;12(5):3115–22.
27. Pestalozzi BC, Zahrieh D, Mallon E, Gusterson BA, Price KN, Gelber RD, et al. Distinct clinical and prognostic features of infiltrating lobular carcinoma of the breast: combined results of 15 International Breast Cancer Study Group clinical trials. J Clin Oncol. 2008;26(18):3006–14.
28. Dossus L, Benusiglio PR. Lobular breast cancer: incidence and genetic and non-genetic risk factors. Breast Cancer Res. 2015;17:37.
29. Shimizu H, Nakayama KI. A 23 gene-based molecular prognostic score precisely predicts overall survival of breast cancer patients. EBioMedicine. 2019;46:150–9.
30. Tappeiner E, Finotello F, Charoentong P, Mayer C, Rieder D, Trajanoski Z. TIminer: NGS data mining pipeline for cancer immunology and immunotherapy. Bioinformatics. 2017;33(19):3140–1.
31. Y-Y Chen Patterns of lobular carcinoma in situ and their diagnostic mimics in core needle biopsies; 2009
32. Watermann DO, Tempfer C, Hefler LA, Parat C, Stickeler E. Ultrasound morphology of invasive lobular breast cancer is different compared with other types of breast cancer. Ultrasound Med Biol. 2005;31(2):167–74.
33. Chapellier C, Balu-Maestro C, Bleuse A, Ettore F, Bruneton JN. Ultrasonography of invasive lobular carcinoma of the breast: sonographic patterns and diagnostic value. Clin Imaging. 2000;24(6):333–6.
34. Brkljacic B, Divjak E, Tomasovic-Loncaric C, Tesic V, Ivanac G. Shear-wave sonoelastographic features of invasive lobular breast cancers. Croat Med J. 2016;57(1):42–50.
35. Selinko VL, Middleton LP, Dempsey PJ. Role of sonography in diagnosing and staging invasive lobular carcinoma. J Clin Ultrasound. 2004;32(7):323–32.
36. Rissanen T et al. Ultrasonography of invasive lobular breast carcinoma; 1998
37. Joycelyn Jie Xin L, Guek EL. A review of invasive lobular carcinoma of the breast: Should it be treated like invasive ductal carcinoma? Integr Cancer Sci Ther. 2016;3(5)
38. Le Gal M, Ollivier L, Asselain B, Meunier M, Laurent M, Vielh P, et al. Mammographic features of 455 invasive lobular carcinomas. Radiology. 1992;185(3):705–8.
39. Wen HY, Brogi E. Lobular carcinoma in situ. Surg Pathol Clin. 2018;11(1):123–45.
40. Mendelson EB, Harris KM, Doshi N, Tobon H. Infiltrating lobular carcinoma: mammographic patterns with pathologic correlation. AJR Am J Roentgenol. 1989;153(2):265–71.
41. Arpino G, Bardou VJ, Clark GM, Elledge RM. Infiltrating lobular carcinoma of the breast: tumor characteristics and clinical outcome. Breast Cancer Res. 2004;6(3):R149–56.
42. Biglia N, Mariani L, Sgro L, Mininanni P, Moggio G, Sismondi P. Increased incidence of lobular breast cancer in women treated with hormone replacement therapy: implications for diagnosis, surgical and medical treatment. Endocr Relat Cancer. 2007;14(3):549–67.
43. de Deus MR, Wludarski SC, Carvalho FM, Bacchi CE. Immunohistochemistry applied to the differential diagnosis between ductal and lobular carcinoma of the breast. Appl Immunohistochem Mol Morphol. 2013;21(1):1–12.
44. Kim SH, Seo BK, Lee J, Kim SJ, Cho KR, Lee KY, et al. Correlation of ultrasound findings with histology, tumor grade, and biological markers in breast cancer. Acta Oncol. 2008;47(8):1531–8.
45. Sneige N, Wang J, Baker BA, Krishnamurthy S, Middleton LP. Clinical, histopathologic, and biologic features of pleomorphic lobular (ductal-lobular) carcinoma in situ of the breast: a report of 24 cases. Mod Pathol. 2002;15(10):1044–50.
46. Kao L, Bulkin Y, Fineberg S, Montgomery L, Koenigsberg T. A case report: lobular carcinoma in situ in a male patient with subsequent invasive ductal carcinoma identified on screening breast MRI. J Cancer. 2012;3:226–30.
47. Haagensen CD et al. Lobular neoplasia (so called lobular carcinoma in situ) of the breast; 1978
48. Langley RR, Fidler IJ. The seed and soil hypothesis revisited – the role of tumor-stroma interactions in metastasis to different organs. Int J Cancer. 2011;128(11):2527–35.

49. Sarkar S, Horn G, Moulton K, Oza A, Byler S, Kokolus S, et al. Cancer development, progression, and therapy: an epigenetic overview. Int J Mol Sci. 2013;14(10):21087–113.
50. Da Costa D, Taddese A, Cure ML, Gerson D, Poppiti R Jr, Esserman LE. Common and unusual diseases of the nipple-areolar complex. Radiographics. 2007;27(Suppl 1):S65–77.
51. Lim B, Woodward WA, Wang X, Reuben JM, Ueno NT. Inflammatory breast cancer biology: the tumour microenvironment is key. Nat Rev Cancer. 2018;18:485–99.
52. Barkana BD, El-Sayed A, Khaled RH, Helal M, Khaled H, Deeb R, et al. Imaging modalities in inflammatory breast cancer (IBC) diagnosis: a computer-aided diagnosis system using bilateral mammography images. Sensors (Basel). 2022;23(1)
53. Alunni JP. Imaging inflammatory breast cancer. Diagn Interv Imaging. 2012;93(2):95–103.
54. Wang L, Wang D, Fei X, Ruan M, Chai W, Xu L, et al. A rim-enhanced mass with central cystic changes on MR imaging: how to distinguish breast cancer from inflammatory breast diseases? PLoS One. 2014;9(3):e90355.
55. Telli ML, Horst KC, Guardino AE, Dirbas FM, Carlson RW. Phyllodes tumors of the breast: natural history, diagnosis, and treatment. J Natl Compr Cancer Netw. 2007;5(3):324–30.
56. Kalambo M, Adrada BE, Adeyefa MM, Krishnamurthy S, Hess K, Carkaci S, et al. Phyllodes tumor of the breast: ultrasound-pathology correlation. AJR Am J Roentgenol. 2018;210(4):W173–W9.

Rare Forms of Breast Cancer

4

Contents

4.1 Adenocarcinoma of the Breast

Breast adenocarcinomas (ADCs) are primarily divided into two main subtypes: infiltrating ductal and infiltrating lobular carcinomas, which share similar clinical features and genetic mutations (see Fig. 4.1). Most breast cancers develop from a background of premalignant changes, progressing in a histological sequence from usual ductal or lobular hyperplasia to atypical hyperplasia, carcinoma in situ, and eventually invasive tumors (see Fig. 4.1). Around 10% of breast cancers are strongly linked to family history and tend to appear in younger women. Through family-based studies, two key breast cancer susceptibility genes have been identified:

K. Malherbe, *A Mammographers Guide: Radiological and Histopathological Guidelines*, https://doi.org/10.1007/978-3-031-84667-0_4

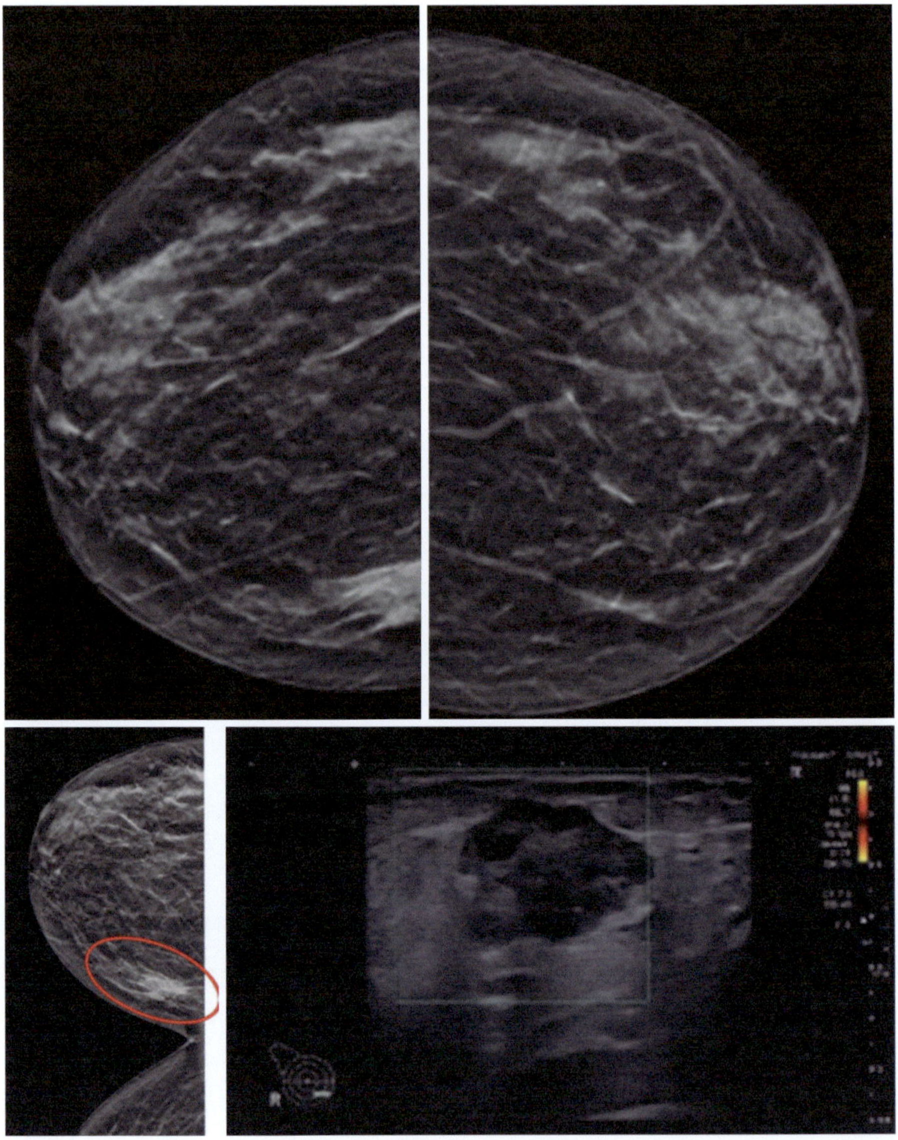

Fig. 4.1 Bilateral mammogram images demonstrating ductal adenocarcinoma of the right breast-Bilateral CC views demonstrated an ill-defined density in the far medial aspect of the right breast, additional cleavage, and XCCM views were done
Ultrasound demonstrated a hypoechoic lobulated mass with extension into the surrounding tissue

BRCA1 on chromosome 17q21 and BRCA2 on chromosome 13q12. Women who carry BRCA1 mutations face an 85–90% lifetime risk of breast cancer and about a 33% risk of ovarian cancer [1, 2].

While BRCA1 and BRCA2 were initially thought to be primarily associated with hereditary cases, recent research suggests that in sporadic (nonfamilial) breast cancers with loss of heterozygosity (LOH) at 17q21, BRCA1 can become inactivated due to promoter hypermethylation of the second allele, indicating a potential broader role of BRCA1 in sporadic cancers. This epigenetic mechanism, similar to the mutations seen in hereditary cases, may prove to be common in sporadic breast cancers. Other significant genetic factors in breast cancer include the tumor suppressor gene p53 and the ATM gene on chromosome 11q23. Individuals with germline p53 mutations, known as Li-Fraumeni syndrome, are at a heightened risk for breast cancer, with about half of sporadic breast cancers also showing p53 mutations. Similarly, patients with ATM mutations have a predisposition to breast cancer, with 40% of sporadic cases showing LOH at the ATM gene locus. The frequency of promoter hypermethylation for ATM in sporadic tumors is still under investigation [1, 2]. Another key oncogene in breast cancer research is Her-2 neu (c-erbB2), which shares similarities with the epidermal growth factor receptor and encodes a transmembrane glycoprotein with tyrosine kinase activity. Her-2 neu amplification is observed in 20–30% of breast cancers, where it correlates strongly with increased tumor growth. Herceptin (trastuzumab), a monoclonal antibody targeting Her-2 neu, has become a notable therapeutic agent, particularly for advanced breast cancer cases that overexpress this oncogene. It has been shown to improve survival rates and slow disease progression, marking a significant achievement in translational cancer research [1, 2].

4.2 Tuberculosis (TB) Carcinoma of the Breast

Breast tuberculosis is a rare condition, even in areas where tuberculosis is common, and is often a diagnostic challenge due to its nonspecific clinical and imaging features. A definitive diagnosis requires identifying the bacilli through microbiological or histopathological analysis. This case involved a 52-year-old woman who presented with a painful lump in her left breast for 2 months (see Fig. 4.2). Imaging initially suggested a breast abscess, and subsequent aspiration of the purulent collection led to a diagnosis of tuberculous mammary abscess using molecular testing (GeneXpert). This case highlights the clinical, radiological, and biological features of breast tuberculosis and emphasizes the value of molecular biology in its rapid diagnosis and management [3–5].

The initial breast ultrasound revealed an ill-defined, hypoechoic, fluid-filled mass in the inner lower quadrant of the left breast, classified as a BIRADS 4 lesion. To further characterize the lesion, a breast MRI was performed, revealing a hyperintense area on T2-weighted images with irregular borders and rim enhancement on post-contrast sequences, consistent with an abscess. No indications of malignancy or abnormal enhancement were observed [3–5]. Ultrasound-guided fine needle

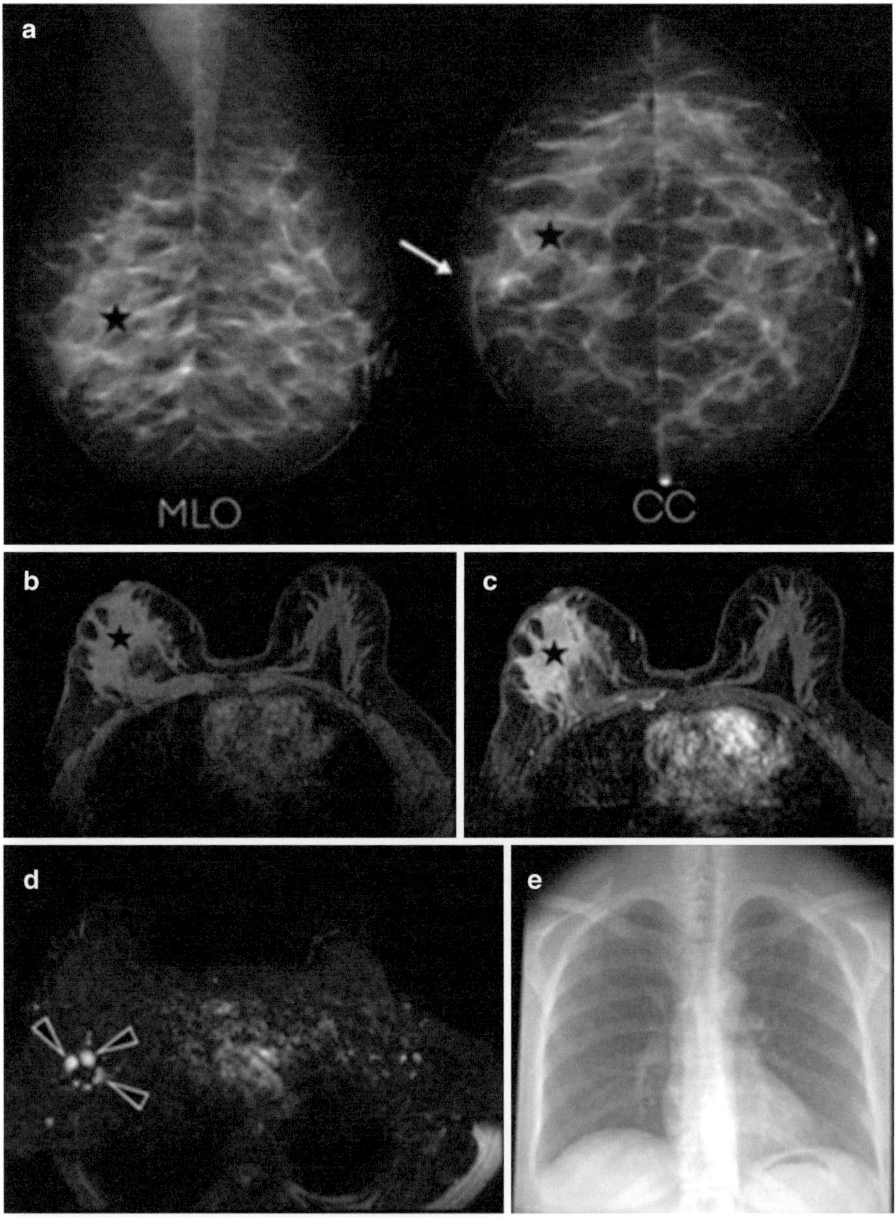

Fig. 4.2 Multimodality imaging of TB carcinoma of the breast [6] Mammograms of a 44-year-old female demonstrate disseminated tuberculosis in right breast (**a**) shows an asymmetric opacity (star) and thickening of the skin (arrow). MRI images of the same patient: pre-contrast fat-suppressed T1-weighted (**b**), post-contrast fat-suppressed T1-weighted (**c**), and fat-suppressed T2-weighted images (**d**) show homogeneous nonmass enhancement with regional type distribution (star) and axillary lymph nodes (arrowheads). The chest x-ray (**e**) of the patient is negative for pulmonary tuberculosis

aspiration yielded 2 mL of bloody, purulent material for cytobacteriological analysis, which showed no cellular reaction or bacterial growth, with both aerobic and anaerobic cultures remaining sterile after 24 hours. Staining techniques (auramine and Ziehl-Neelsen) identified acid-fast bacilli, and GeneXpert testing confirmed *Mycobacterium tuberculosis* presence without rifampin resistance. Further cultures on solid Lowenstein-Jensen medium and liquid MGIT confirmed M. tuberculosis growth within 25 and 13 days, respectively. Given the purulent nature of the sample, an anatomical pathology examination was not conducted [3–5].

A thoracic CT scan revealed no abnormalities. However, histological analysis later demonstrated a granulomatous lesion with caseating granuloma, containing multinucleated Langhans giant cells and epithelioid histiocytes, confirming tuberculosis mastitis. Remarkably, there was also evidence of high-grade ductal carcinoma in situ (DCIS) with an invasive component, highlighting the complex nature of this case. Special Ziehl-Neelsen staining confirmed the presence of acid-fast bacilli within macrophages, solidifying the diagnosis of tuberculosis mastitis [3–5].

Breast tuberculosis remains challenging to diagnose, as imaging modalities like mammography and ultrasound often yield findings similar to breast cancer, making it hard to distinguish between the two [3–5]. Advanced imaging tools, such as CT and MRI, help define the lesion's extent but are limited in diagnostic specificity. In a few cases, a chest X-ray may show signs of active or healed lung tuberculosis or axillary lymph node calcifications. Mammography in breast tuberculosis can reveal masses with ill-defined borders, stromal coarseness, asymmetric density, or nipple retraction, while ultrasound may show heterogeneous masses that can mimic cysts or abscesses. In cases with dense breast tissue, ultrasound aids in detecting masses obscured by mammography (see Fig. 4.3). Axillary lymphadenopathy is commonly found in chronic tuberculosis mastitis, with ultrasound helping to identify lymph nodes with benign features [3–5].

CT scans may be useful for assessing thoracic wall involvement in patients with deeply adherent breast lumps, and MRI can reveal abscess-like signals but is primarily helpful in identifying the lesion's extramammary spread. Confirming breast tuberculosis requires cytology, showing granulomas, Langhans giant cells, and lymphohistiocytic aggregates, typically obtained through core needle biopsy or, in some cases, open biopsy of suspicious areas [3–5]. Staining for acid-fast bacilli (AFB) is often negative but remains an essential part of diagnosis in persistent cases. Fine needle aspiration and cytology (FNAC) are valuable for diagnosing breast tuberculosis, with reported success rates up to 100% when granulomas and necrosis are present [3–5].

Polymerase chain reaction (PCR) tests offer a sensitive method for detecting tuberculosis in breast tissue, especially in culture-negative cases, although false positives are possible [3–5]. Treatment decisions for breast tuberculosis with coexistent cancer rely on the TNM staging system, but tuberculosis involvement can sometimes exaggerate tumor size, potentially reducing breast conservation options. In such cases, radical mastectomy is generally followed by antitubercular treatment (ATT) for 6–12 months. The standard ATT regimen includes an initial two-month intensive phase with four drugs (ethambutol, pyrazinamide, rifampicin, isoniazid)

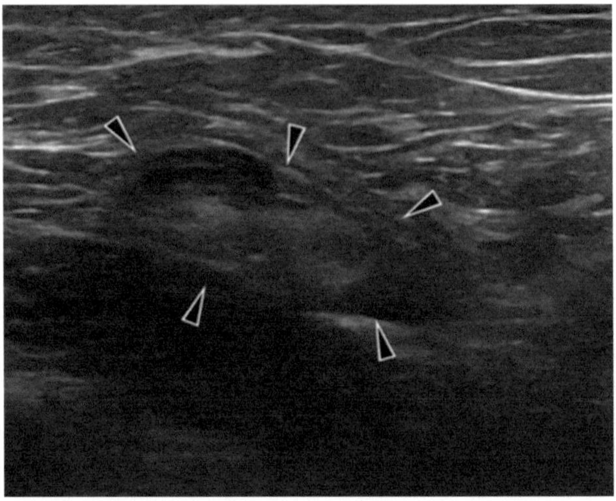

Fig. 4.3 Ultrasound image of TB carcinoma of the breast
Ultrasound image of a 34-year-old female patient (she had a recently developed clinically suspicious palpable lesion) diagnosed with breast tuberculosis demonstrates nodular tuberculosis (arrowheads). The mass is observed as a well-circumscribed, oval-shaped, heterogeneous solid lesion [6]

and a four-month continuation phase with isoniazid and rifampicin. For cases of breast tuberculosis without associated cancer, minimal surgical interventions such as abscess drainage or sinus scraping are generally sufficient, with mastectomy reserved for extensive disease that precludes organ preservation [3–5].

4.3 Myofibroblastoma

Myofibroblastoma is a rare benign spindle cell tumor of the breast, more frequently seen in men but also occurring in women. First described in 1987, it can be challenging for pathologists to distinguish from malignant lesions on biopsy, often requiring surgical excision for confirmation. Clinically, it presents as a solid, mobile mass, with histology showing well-circumscribed fascicles of spindle-shaped cells interspersed with adipocytes in a collagenous background. Imaging, such as mammography and ultrasound, often reveals a round, well-defined mass, which may resemble other benign conditions like spindle cell lipoma. Although uncommon, myofibroblastoma can also occur along the milk line or in extramammary sites [7, 8].

The tumor cells are positive for CD34, vimentin, and estrogen receptors, among other markers, and negative for markers like CD117 and S100, reflecting its fibroblastic origin. On MRI, myofibroblastoma often shows a homogeneously enhanced, circumscribed mass with high signal intensity on T2-weighted images, helping distinguish it from malignant lesions through diffusion-weighted imaging. Fine needle aspiration or core needle biopsy can be performed for diagnosis, though core biopsy is more reliable due to limited cellularity in fine needle samples (see Figs. 4.4 and 4.5) [7, 8].

Treatment involves surgical excision primarily for symptom relief, with no documented cases of malignancy or recurrence, though follow-up is recommended for at least 24 months. Long-term stability of untreated cases remains unclear, as almost all reported cases have undergone excision [7, 8].

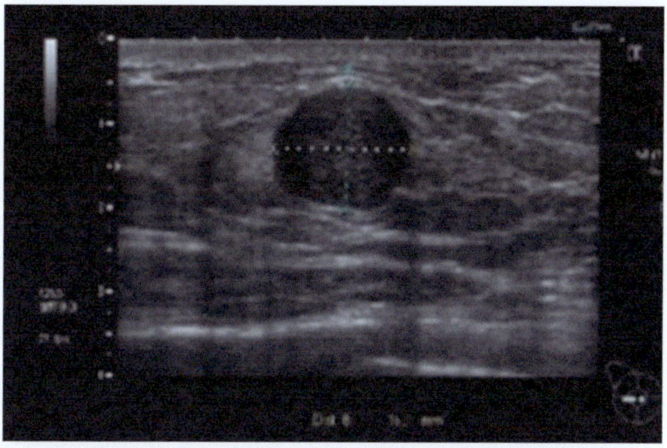

Fig. 4.4 Case study of myofibroblastoma of the breast [9]

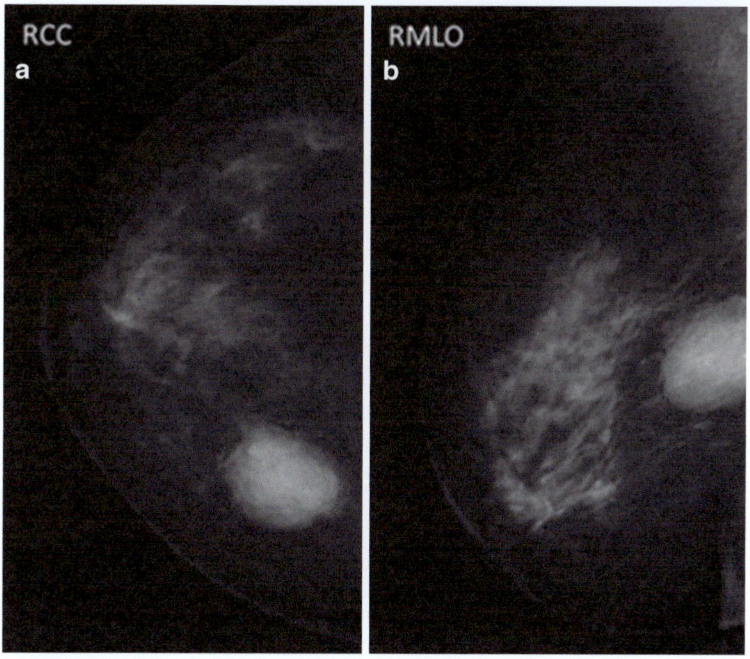

Fig. 4.5 Mammographic imaging of a myofibroblastoma in the right breast, presenting as a dense, lobulated mass in the inner medial quadrant of the breast [10]

4.4 Angiosarcoma

Angiosarcoma (AS) of the breast is an uncommon tumor, representing only about 1% of all soft tissue breast tumors [11]. It can present as a primary tumor, usually in women aged 30–50, or as a secondary tumor typically associated with prior radiotherapy, especially in women with a median age of 67–71 years. Primary AS arises in the breast tissue and sometimes involves the skin, accounting for less than 0.04% of all malignant neoplasms. In contrast, secondary AS often appears around 10 years after radiation therapy for breast cancer, with studies suggesting an increased risk following doses of radiation above 50 Gy [11]. AS linked with chronic lymphedema outside a radiation field, particularly in a limb after mastectomy and radiotherapy, is known as Stewart-Treves syndrome [11].

Diagnostic imaging for AS, such as mammograms and ultrasounds, often lacks distinguishing features, leading to possible misclassification as benign, particularly in younger women. MRI, however, has shown utility in identifying malignancy patterns with AS, often presenting as hyperintense on T2-weighted images with rapid contrast washout (see Fig. 4.7). Fine needle aspiration (FNA) or core needle biopsy (CNB) is typically used for diagnosis, with excessive bleeding during FNA potentially indicating the highly vascular nature of AS. Histopathology reveals irregular vascular formations with hyperchromatic nuclei, and immunohistologic staining for endothelial markers like CD31 confirms the diagnosis (see Figs. 4.6 and 4.7) [11]. There is no consensus on optimal surgical management for AS, although mastectomy is commonly performed for primary cases, and wide local excision is used in secondary cases, though the depth of resection is debated. Given the aggressiveness of AS, treatment is often multidisciplinary, involving surgical, medical, and

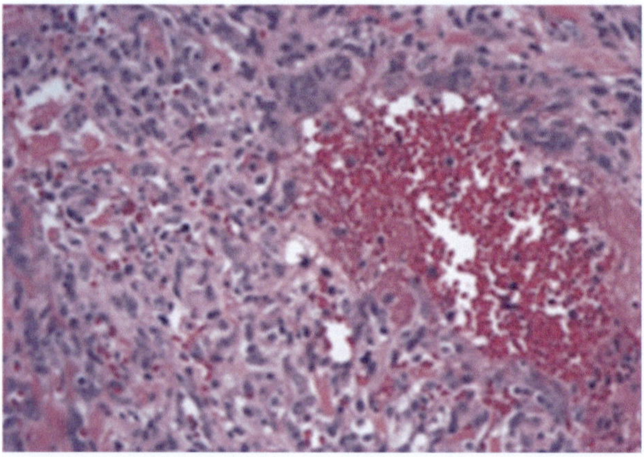

Fig. 4.6 Primary angiosarcoma of the breast on histology
One specific pathological feature of a radiation-induced breast angiosarcoma is a so-called blood lakes which are pools of extravasated erythrocytes. Other characteristics of RIBA tumors are clear necrosis, mitotic activity, solid and spindle cell foci, papillary formations, endothelial tufting, and well-marked endothelial cell atypic

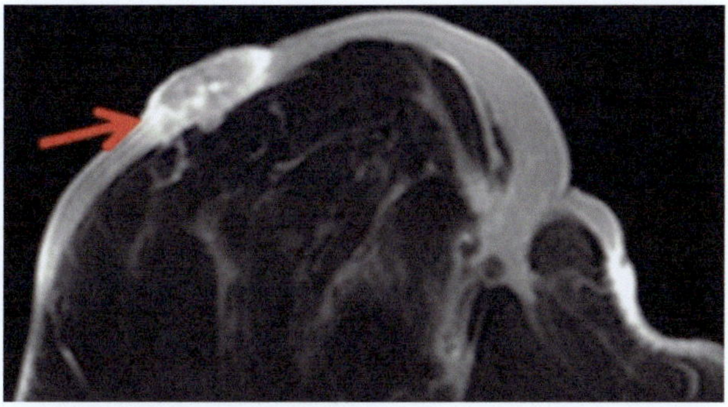

Fig. 4.7 Angiosarcoma as demonstrated with MRI imaging
Overall skin thickening is noted with a high signal along the thickened area within the subcutaneous soft tissue of the breast

radiation oncology specialists. While aggressive surgical intervention is generally recommended, the roles of neoadjuvant or adjuvant therapies remain undefined, emphasizing the importance of specialized care for this complex malignancy [11].

Unique Imaging Features of Angiosarcoma of the Breast

- Mammography typically detects a noncalcified, ill-defined mass or focal or growing asymmetry, and however it might be unrevealing.
- Ultrasound frequently shows a mixed hyper and hypoechoic ill-defined lesion, which was previously characterized as relatively specific to PBA and particularly common in larger lesions.
- Angiosarcoma can also manifest as a hypo- or hyperechoic mass, with the latter being associated with benign entities such as fat-containing lesions and fibrosis.
- Doppler can be decisive in this context, identifying low-resistance flow [11].

4.5 Male Breast Cancer

Male breast cancer is rare, accounting for only 0.2% of all male malignancies. A 20-year national registry analysis of surgically removed breast specimens with gynecomastia found a 0.11% overall frequency of invasive carcinomas and 0.18% of in situ carcinomas [12–26]. Although male breast cancer is uncommon and gynecomastia is not regarded as a premalignant condition, men with gynecomastia, particularly the elderly, are concerned about breast cancer and frequently seek medical counsel; therefore it is critical to distinguish male breast cancer from gynecomastia (see Fig. 4.8). Men with Klinefelter syndrome are 20- to 50-fold more likely to develop breast cancer. Other risk factors include obesity, alcohol, exogenous estrogen exposure (such as gender reassignment), and testicular problems [12–26].

It is uncertain if these are breast cancer-specific concerns associated with the stimulatory process that causes gynecomastia. Old age, working in a

Fig. 4.8 Bilateral MLO images of a male breast Images demonstrating a dense hypoechoic mass in the prepectoral space of the left breast

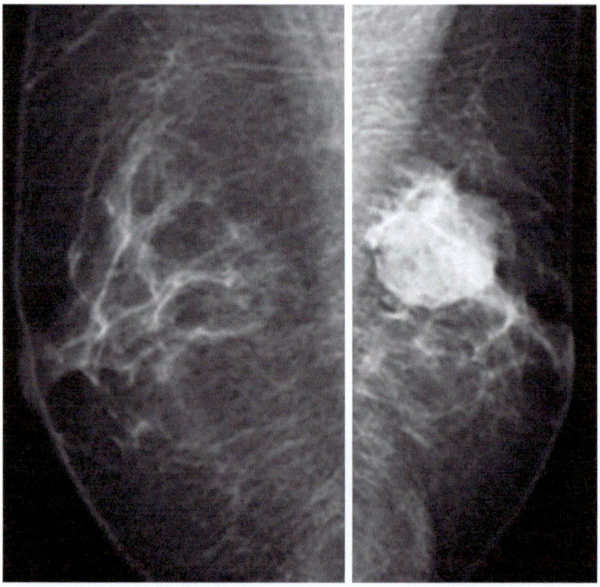

Table 4.1 Clinical findings of gynecomastia and male breast cancer

Clinical findings	Gynecomastia	Male breast cancer
Unilateral/ bilateral	Mostly bilateral, can be unilateral	Unilateral
Consistency	Rubbery or firm	Firm or hard
Location	Concentric, around the nipple	More peripheral, outside the nipple
Pain	Painful if recent onset or rapid enlargement	Usually painless
Associated features such as skin dimpling, nipple retraction, bloody discharge	No	Possible
Palpable axillary or supraclavicular lymph node(s)	No	Possible

high-temperature environment, exhaust fumes, chest radiation, and liver damage are all risk factors for male breast cancer. Family history should always be investigated. For instance, a family history of BRCA2 positive breast cancer considerably raises the risk of male breast cancer among mutation carriers (see Table 4.1) [12–26].

4.5.1 Prevention of Gynecomastia in Men with Prostate Cancer

Because androgen deprivation is a typical treatment for advanced prostate cancer, doctors are particularly concerned about its role in the development of gynecomastia. Gynecomastia can develop in up to 80% of patients following nonsteroidal antiandrogen medication, typically 6–9 months after hormonal treatment. Some patients may get painful and disfiguring gynecomastia. Tamoxifen, radiation treatment, and aromatase inhibitors are all viable preventive strategies [12–26].

Tamoxifen is the most effective preventive medicine for gynecomastia as an antiandrogen therapy for prostate cancer. A randomized controlled trial found that tamoxifen is more effective than radiation in preventing gynecomastia in patients receiving bicalutamide (Casodex) for prostate cancer. Tamoxifen is more effective than aromatase inhibitors at preventing gynecomastia in prostate cancer patients [12–26].

According to current evidence, tamoxifen 10–20 mg per day is the optimal dose for preventing gynecomastia in prostate cancer patients following androgen deprivation therapy. Low-dose prophylactic irradiation has been shown to minimize the incidence of gynecomastia but not breast discomfort in males using estrogens or antiandrogens for prostate cancer. Irradiation appears to be less effective than tamoxifen in the prevention and treatment of gynecomastia, but it is often well tolerated [12–26].

Some studies suggest that the current generation of antiandrogen medicines such as abiraterone acetate, enzalutamide, apalutamide, and darolutamide could be related with decreased gynecomastia. More recently, it has been reported that 36.6% of individuals receiving enzalutamide develop gynecomastia, but this prevalence appears to be reduced [12–26].

Imaging Guidelines for Male Breast

- Asymptomatic or symptomatic.
- Personal history of breast or prostate cancer.
- Family history of breast or prostate cancer.
- BRCA 1 or BRCA 2 gene mutation positive.

4.6 Paget's Disease

4.6.1 Introduction

Paget disease of the breast (also known as Paget disease of the nipple or mammary Paget disease) is a rare type of cancer that affects the skin of the nipple and, in most cases, the darker circle of skin around it known as the areola. The majority of persons with Paget disease of the breast have one or more tumors within the same breast. These tumors are either invasive breast cancer or ductal carcinoma in situ [27–29].

Paget disease of the breast is named after Sir James Paget, a nineteenth century British clinician who, in 1874, discovered a link between nipple alterations and breast cancer. (Several other disorders bear Sir James Paget's name, including bone Paget disease and extramammary Paget disease, which includes vulvar and penile Paget disease [27–29].

Paget cells, or malignant cells, are a telltale symptom of Paget illness in the breast. These cells can be found in the epidermis (surface layer) of the skin on the nipple and areola. Under a microscope, Paget cells frequently seem big and spherical; they can be seen as solitary cells or in small groups within the epidermis [27–29].

Paget disease of the breast affects both men and women; however women account for the majority of cases. Paget disease of the breast occurs in around 1–4% of all breast cancer cases. The typical age of diagnosis is 57 years, but the condition has been discovered in teens and persons in their late 80s [27–29].

4.6.2 Pathophysiology and Histopathology

The most widely recognized explanation holds that cancer cells from a tumor in the breast move down the milk ducts to the nipple and areola. This would explain why Paget disease and malignancies within the same breast are usually frequently discovered together. A second idea proposes that cells in the nipple or areola develop cancer on their own. This could explain why some patients develop Paget disease of the breast without having a tumor in the same breast. Furthermore, it is possible that Paget disease and malignancies inside the same breast develop separately [27–29].

Paget's disease (PD) is a rare cutaneous intraepithelial malignancy characterized by large adenocarcinoma cells with copious mucin. It is classified into two subgroups based on the affected anatomic location: mammary Paget's disease (MPD) and extramammary Paget's disease (EMPD). Epidemiologically, MPD accounts for 1–4.3% of all primary breast carcinoma, with 93–100% of MPD related with underlying ductal carcinoma of the breast, whereas EMPD typically affects apocrine gland-bearing sites, such as the vulva in females (81.3%) and the scrotum in males (43.2%). Since 1978, the incidence of EMPD has increased with an annual percent change of +3.2%, with scrotum EMPD accounting for 21% of primary scrotal carcinomas. Interestingly, the EMPD afflicted organs typically involve the vulva in females and the scrotum in males, which are hormonally targeted tissues [27–29].

Although vulvar EMPD is uncommon, some studies have reported heterochronous development of EMPD in the vulva and MPD, as well as synchronous development of EMPD in the vulva and MPD lesions. Furthermore, the performance status of a patient with ER-positive EMPD was preserved after treatment with the ER inhibitor tamoxifen. This successful data indicates that hormone therapy could be an option for some cases of advanced EMPD [10]. As a result, hormone receptors may serve as a link between MPD and EMPD, providing insight into their similar etiology [27–29].

4.6.3 Clinical Evaluation and Imaging

The symptoms of Paget disease in the breast are sometimes confused with those of benign skin disorders such as dermatitis or eczema [27–29].

These symptoms could include the following:

- Itching, tingling, or redness in the nipple or areola.
- Flaky, crusty, or thicker skin on or around the nipple (see Fig. 4.9).
- A flat nipple.
- Yellowish or reddish nipple discharge [27–29]

Because the early signs of Paget disease of the breast may resemble a benign skin condition, and the disease is uncommon, it is often misdiagnosed at first. People with Paget disease of the breast frequently experience symptoms for several months before being properly diagnosed [27–29].

- A nipple biopsy enables doctors to accurately detect Paget disease of the breast. There are various forms of nipple biopsy, including those mentioned here.
- Surface biopsy is the process of delicately scraping cells from the skin's surface using a glass slide or other equipment.
- Shave biopsy: The skin's top layer is removed using a razor-like tool.
- A punch biopsy involves the removal of a disk-shaped sample of tissue using a circular cutting tool known as a punch. Wedge biopsy: A scalpel is used to cut out a small wedge of tissue [27–29].

In some circumstances, doctors may extract the entire nipple. A pathologist then analyzes the cells or tissue using a microscope to look for Paget cells [27–29].

Most persons with Paget disease of the breast have one or more tumors within the same breast. In addition to scheduling a nipple biopsy, the doctor should conduct a clinical breast exam to look for lumps or other abnormalities. Up to 50% of persons with Paget disease of the breast have a breast lump that may be felt during a clinical breast examination. To screen for potential cancers, the doctor may request additional diagnostic procedures such as a diagnostic mammography, ultrasound exam, or magnetic resonance imaging scan (see Figs. 4.10 and 4.11) [27–29].

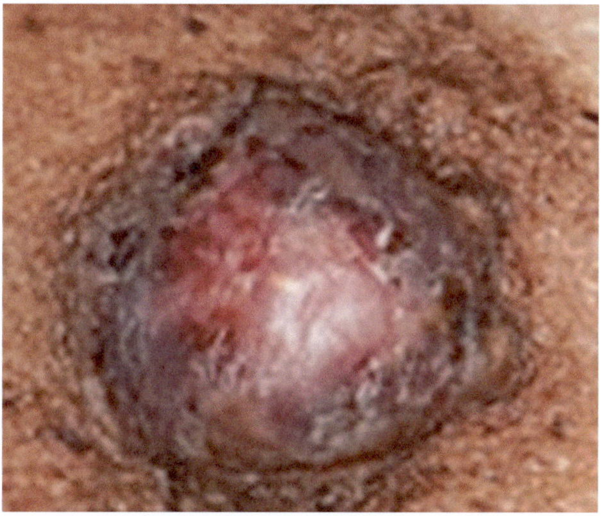

Fig. 4.9 Clinical appearance of Paget's disease of the nipple

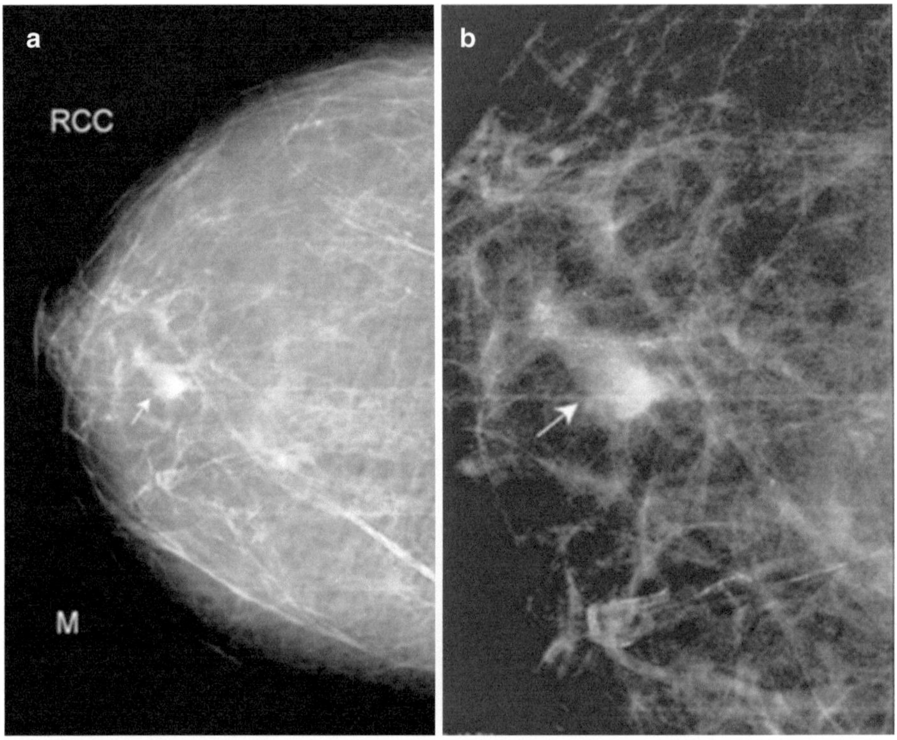

Fig. 4.10 Right CC mammogram and B-Mode ultrasound image of Paget's disease of the breast [30]
A 71-year-old female came with a complaint of itching and eczema around the right nipple with a history of nipple discharge. There was no mass palpable on clinical examination. Mammogram of the right breast showed an asymmetric density (arrow) in the cranio-caudal (CC) view (**a** and **b**) that was not seen on ultrasound. The patient underwent a simple mastectomy. Histopathology showed features of Paget's disease of the nipple with invasive ductal carcinoma grade 2

4.6.4 Treatment and Management

For many years, mastectomy, with or without the removal of lymph nodes under the arm on the same side of the chest (known as axillary lymph node dissection), was considered the usual procedure for Paget disease of the breast. This sort of surgery was performed because individuals with Paget disease of the breast were virtually usually discovered to have one or more tumors within the same breast. Even if just one tumor was present, it could be several centimeters away from the nipple and areola, rendering surgery on the nipple and areola ineffective [27–29].

However, studies have shown that breast-conserving surgery that includes the removal of the nipple and areola, followed by whole-breast radiation therapy, is a

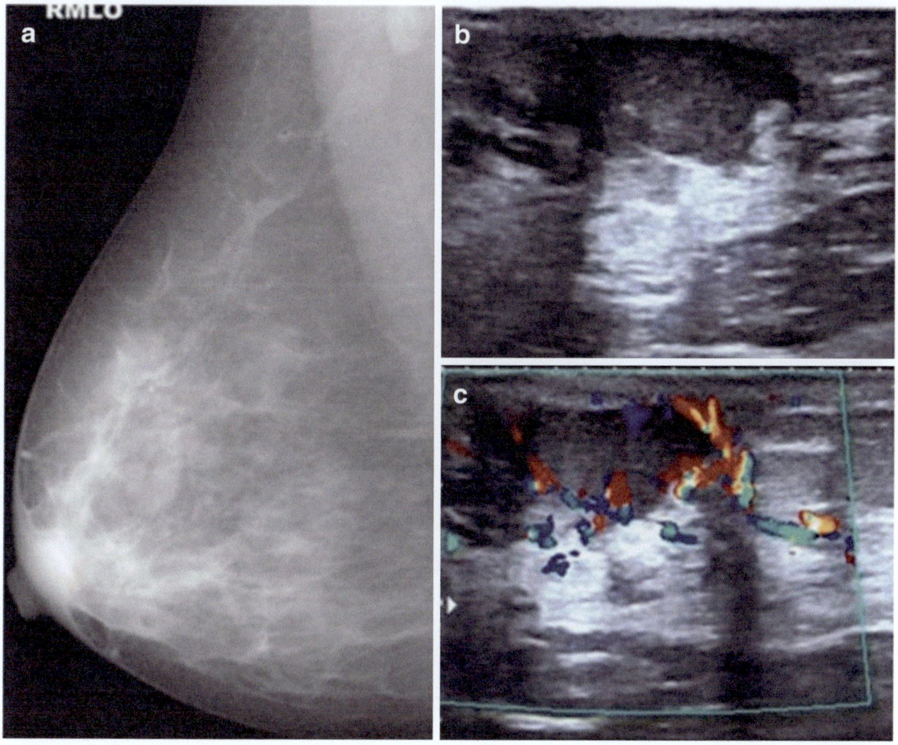

Fig. 4.11 Right MLO mammogram and ultrasound image of Paget's disease A 51-year-old female presented with a lump in the right nipple–areolar region of 3 months' duration with an off-and-on history of nipple discharge. No history of fever was present. Mammogram of the right breast, MLO view (**a**), shows diffuse thickening in the nipple areolar region; however, no microcalcifications are seen. Ultrasound of the right breast (**b**) shows a well-defined hypoechoic lesion in the nipple areolar region with peripheral vascularity (**c**) on color Doppler

safe option for people with Paget disease of the breast who do not have a palpable lump in their breast and whose mammograms do not reveal a tumor. People with Paget disease of the breast who have a breast tumor and are undergoing mastectomy should be offered a sentinel lymph node biopsy to determine whether the malignancy has progressed to the axillary lymph nodes [27–29]. If cancer cells are discovered in the sentinel lymph node(s), extensive axillary lymph node surgery may be required [27–29].

Adjuvant therapy, consisting of chemotherapy and/or hormonal therapy, may also be recommended depending on the stage and other characteristics of the underlying breast tumor (for example, the presence or absence of lymph node involvement, estrogen and progesterone receptors in tumor cells, and HER2 protein overexpression in tumor cells) [27–29].

4.7 Mucinous Carcinoma

4.7.1 Introduction

Mucinous carcinoma of the breast is an uncommon subtype of breast cancer, accounting for only around 2% of all breast carcinomas [1, 31, 32]. According to the most recent WHO classification of breast cancers, mucinous carcinoma is a distinct kind of breast cancer. Mucinous carcinomas are classified into two categories based on their cellularity:

- The pure type mucinous carcinoma.
- The mixed type mucinous carcinoma [1, 31, 32].

The pure variety is entirely composed of tumor tissue, with extracellular mucin produced in more than 90% of the tumor, whereas the mixed form includes an infiltrating ductal epithelial component that lacks mucin. Mucinous breast cancer has a good prognosis, with a low recurrence rate and a low risk of lymph node metastases. Histopathological examination is the primary method for making a definitive diagnosis and classifying mucinous breast carcinomas [1, 31, 32].

4.7.2 Pathophysiology and Histopathology

Transcriptomic investigations have revealed that mucinous tumors are of luminal A molecular subtype. The transcriptome aspects of mucinous A tumors differ from those of mucinous B tumors, which exhibit a gene expression pattern comparable to neuroendocrine carcinoma. Pure mucinous carcinomas have modest levels of genetic instability and uncommon recurrent amplifications, but the genomic profiles of mixed mucinous tumor components are strikingly comparable to those of pure mucinous carcinomas. Diploid cells make up more than 90% of pure mucinous carcinomas, but only 42% of mixed mucinous carcinomas [1, 31, 32].

A gross anatomical examination of mucinous carcinoma of the breast reveals a glistening gelatinous tumor with pushing borders and a distinctive soft consistency. The tumor sizes range from less than 1 cm to more than 20 cm (mean = 3 cm) [1, 31, 32]. Mucinous carcinoma is distinguished histologically by nests of cells floating in lakes of mucin, which are separated by fine fibrous septae carrying capillary blood veins. The cell clusters vary in shape and size, with the occasional tubular arrangement. Although nuclear atypia is uncommon in classic mucinous carcinoma, it might occur in rare situations [1, 31, 32].

A micropapillary or cribriform intraepithelial component is extremely unusual. Mucinous carcinoma with large cell clusters, also known as hypercellular or type B mucinous carcinoma, frequently exhibits neuroendocrine differentiation. Type A mucinous carcinoma, which contains more extracellular mucin, is the classic non-endocrine variant. Pure and mixed forms have been reported. The most prevalent mixing is with aggressive cancer of no particular type [1, 31, 32]. A pure tumor must consist of more than 90% mucinous carcinoma. The in situ component could have a papillary, micropapillary, or cribriform pattern. In rare circumstances, in situ cancer may produce a lot of luminal mucin. Immunohistochemistry and specific stains are sometimes used to detect neuroendocrine differentiation (Grimelius).

Mucinous carcinoma is often positive for estrogen and progesterone receptors, with modest expression of androgen receptors and no HER2 amplification. Pure and mixed mucinous carcinomas have been shown to express WT. Mucinous breast cancer primarily expresses MUC2 and MUC6 from the MUC gene family [1, 31, 32].

4.7.3 Clinical Evaluation and Imaging

Mucinous carcinoma often grows slowly and can reach a significant size upon diagnosis. This is explained by the fact that the tumor's mucinous material does not feel firm or solid under examination. Most individuals with mucinous breast cancer have a palpable breast tumor [1, 31, 32]. Fixation to the skin or chest wall is uncommon but has been recorded in big lesions. With broad screening, many patients are diagnosed with mammographic abnormalities. Circumscribed and lobulated breast lesions are common mammographic findings for mucinous cancer (see Figs. 4.12, 4.13, and 4.14) [1, 31, 32].

A well-defined margin would support the diagnosis of pure mucinous cancer. Mucinous carcinoma appears on ultrasonography as a complicated mass with cystic and solid components, such as microlobulation, vascularity, and distal enhancement. The histologic subtype of mucinous carcinoma can be predicted using echogenicity. Mixed mucinous carcinoma has hypoechoic masses, while pure mucinous carcinoma has isoechoic masses. Mucinous carcinoma appears on an MRI as a lobular form with rim or heterogeneous enhancement, a persistent pattern on the time-intensity curve, and homogenous significantly high signal intensity on T2-weighted images [1, 31, 32].

Differential Diagnoses for Mucinous Carcinoma Include

- Mucocele-like lesion.
- Metastatic mucinous carcinoma.
- Myxomatous fibroadenoma.

4.7.4 Treatment and Management

Mucinous breast cancer is treated with surgery and postoperative hormone therapy in hormone-responsive (estrogen/progesterone) tumors [1, 31, 32]. A new study advocated axillary staging for mucinous cancer using sentinel lymph node biopsy and adjuvant radiation and hormone therapy following breast conserving. Trastuzumab is not used to treat mucinous carcinomas since most of them do not express the HER2/neu protein [1, 31, 32]. Trastuzumab is licensed for the treatment

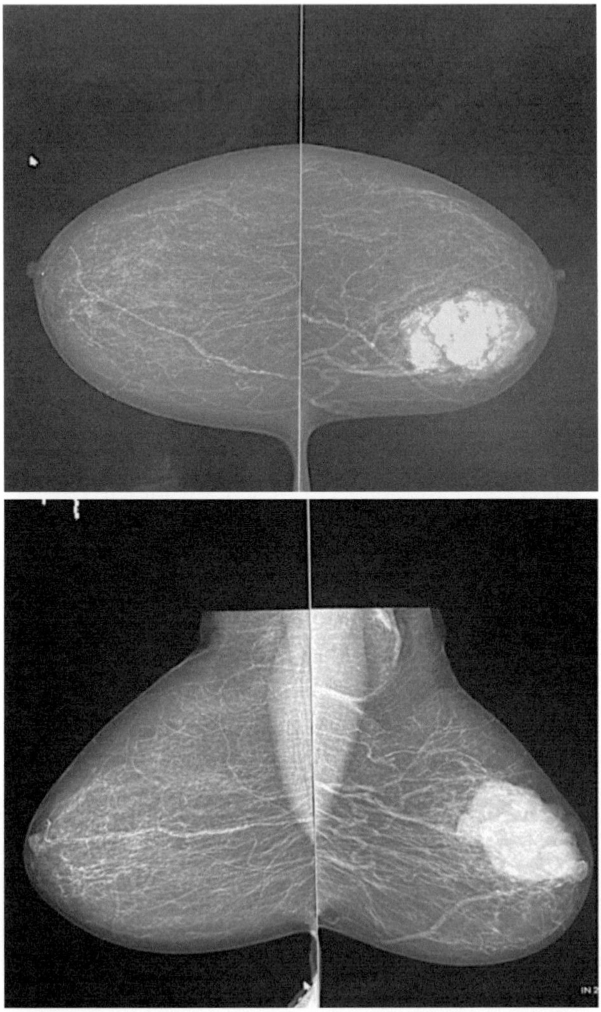

Fig. 4.12 Mammographic appearance of mucinous carcinoma
A 61-year-old female presented with an enlarging left breast lump over a span of 2 years. Left breast on mammogram demonstrated a dense, lobulated mass with extension into the surrounding soft tissue

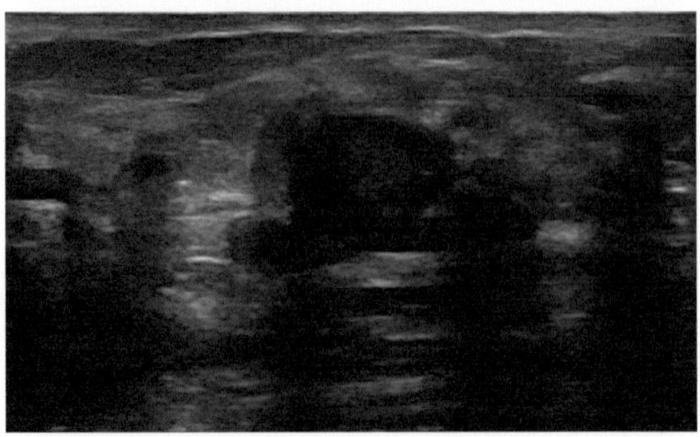

Fig. 4.13 Ultrasound appearance of mucinous carcinoma
A large mass with internal cystic necrosis and vascularity on Power Doppler imaging was noted, in the axilla, there were reactive lymph nodes with loss of central fatty hilum and a hypoechoic appearance

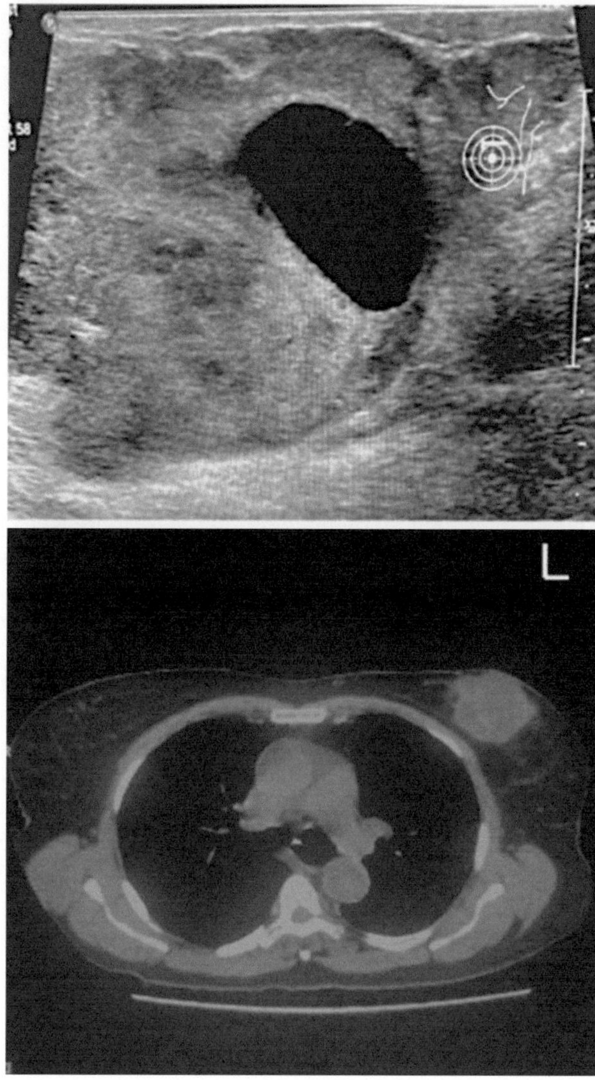

Fig. 4.14 Ultrasound and CT scan image of mucinous carcinoma. CT scan on the right demonstrated a lobulated heterogeneous mass within the left breast with a hypodense center and hyperdense rim and some enhancement post-contrast administration. A few small satellite lesions were noted along the overlying dermis

of metastatic breast cancer as well as adjuvant therapy for early-stage HER2-positive malignancies. Mucinous breast cancer is treated with surgery and postoperative hormone therapy in hormone-responsive (estrogen/progesterone) tumors. A previous study advocated axillary staging for mucinous cancer using sentinel lymph node biopsy and adjuvant radiation and hormone therapy following breast conserving. Trastuzumab is not used to treat mucinous carcinomas since most of them do not express the HER2/neu protein. Trastuzumab is licensed for the treatment of metastatic breast cancer as well as adjuvant therapy for early-stage HER2-positive malignancies [1, 31, 32].

The following considerations may influence treatment decisions:

- Tumor Biology: Because mucinous carcinoma is more common in the elderly, estrogen and progesterone receptors are expressed more frequently than in younger women. Similarly, there are fewer cases of HER-2 overexpression. This influences the choice of appropriate therapy.
- General Health Status: The higher prevalence of comorbidities, frailty, and cognitive decline in senior people are regarded as limiting considerations for selecting treatment.
- Functional status refers to the ability to complete ordinary everyday duties. Functional restriction is independently connected with a lower life expectancy, determining the overall survival of patients.
- The Comprehensive Geriatric Assessment (GCA) can be used to assess older people and improve mucinous carcinoma treatment [1, 31, 32].

4.8 Conclusion

This chapter focused on uncommon types of breast cancer, exploring their unique characteristics, diagnosis, and treatment strategies. The chapter begins with adenocarcinoma of the breast, discussing its cellular makeup and clinical implications. Myofibroblastoma, a rare benign tumor, is examined in terms of its presentation and differentiation from other breast cancers. Angiosarcoma, a malignancy originating from blood vessels, is highlighted for its aggressive nature and diagnostic challenges.

The chapter also covers tuberculosis-associated breast carcinoma (TB breast carcinoma), an unusual form influenced by infectious pathology, and male breast carcinoma, emphasizing the unique clinical considerations and treatment approaches for breast cancer in men. Each section provides an overview of the disease's pathology, diagnostic processes, and therapeutic options, aiming to enhance understanding of these rare conditions. The chapter concludes with a summary, followed by a list of references to support further research on these rare breast cancer types.

References

1. Luna-Abanto J, Mendoza TG. Mucinous carcinoma of the breast: a case report and review of the literature. Medwave. 2017;17(6):e7003.
2. Gazdar AF, Hirsch FR, Minna JD. From mice to men and back: an assessment of preclinical model systems for the study of lung cancers. J Thorac Oncol. 2016;11(3):287–99.
3. Hagen-Ansert SL. Textbook of diagnostic ultrasonography. 2nd ed; 2014.
4. Oucharqui S, Adil H, Benaissa E, Bssaibis F, En-Nafaa I, Maleb A, et al. Breast tuberculosis: a forgotten diagnosis. IDCases. 2021;26:e01341.
5. Bahcecioglu G, Basara G, Ellis BW, Ren X, Zorlutuna P. Breast cancer models: engineering the tumor microenvironment. Acta Biomater. 2020;106:1–21.
6. Baykan AH, Sayiner HS, Inan I, Aydin E, Erturk SM. Primary breast tuberculosis: imaging findings of a rare disease. Insights Imaging. 2021;12(1):19.

7. Orimo A, Gupta PB, Sgroi DC, Arenzana-Seisdedos F, Delaunay T, Naeem R, et al. Stromal fibroblasts present in invasive human breast carcinomas promote tumor growth and angiogenesis through elevated SDF-1/CXCL12 secretion. Cell. 2005;121(3):335–48.
8. Allinen M, Beroukhim R, Cai L, Brennan C, Lahti-Domenici J, Huang H, et al. Molecular characterization of the tumor microenvironment in breast cancer. Cancer Cell. 2004;6(1):17–32.
9. Wargotz ES, Weiss SW, Norris HJ. Myofibroblastoma of the breast. sixteen cases of a distinctive benign mesenchymal tumor. Am J Surg Pathol. 1987;11(7):493–502.
10. Wei L, Jiang G, Bai L, Li T, Ma X, Jiang L, et al. Inflammatory Myofibroblastoma of the breast: a case report. Front Oncol. 2021;11:646336.
11. Arora TK, Terracina KP, Soong J, Idowu MO, Takabe K. Primary and secondary angiosarcoma of the breast. Gland Surg. 2014;3(1):28.
12. Watermann DO, Tempfer C, Hefler LA, Parat C, Stickeler E. Ultrasound morphology of invasive lobular breast cancer is different compared with other types of breast cancer. Ultrasound Med Biol. 2005;31(2):167–74.
13. Izumori A, Takebe K, Sato A. Ultrasound findings and histological features of ductal carcinoma in situ detected by ultrasound examination alone. Breast Cancer. 2010;17(2):136–41.
14. Pestalozzi BC, Zahrieh D, Mallon E, Gusterson BA, Price KN, Gelber RD, et al. Distinct clinical and prognostic features of infiltrating lobular carcinoma of the breast: combined results of 15 international breast cancer study group clinical trials. J Clin Oncol. 2008;26(18):3006–14.
15. Kim SH, Seo BK, Lee J, Kim SJ, Cho KR, Lee KY, et al. Correlation of ultrasound findings with histology, tumor grade, and biological markers in breast cancer. Acta Oncol. 2008;47(8):1531–8.
16. Dromain C, Balleyguier C, Adler G, Garbay JR, Delaloge S. Contrast-enhanced digital mammography. Eur J Radiol. 2009;69(1):34–42.
17. Shan J, Alam SK, Garra B, Zhang Y, Ahmed T. Computer-aided diagnosis for breast ultrasound using computerized BI-RADS features and machine learning methods. Ultrasound Med Biol. 2016;42(4):980–8.
18. Chen DR, Chien CL, Kuo YF. Computer-aided assessment of tumor grade for breast cancer in ultrasound images. Comput Math Methods Med. 2015;2015:914091.
19. Leong AS, Zhuang Z. The changing role of pathology in breast cancer diagnosis and treatment. Pathobiology. 2011;78(2):99–114.
20. Kao L, Bulkin Y, Fineberg S, Montgomery L, Koenigsberg T. A case report: lobular carcinoma in situ in a male patient with subsequent invasive ductal carcinoma identified on screening breast MRI. J Cancer. 2012;3:226–30.
21. Lane DS, Smith RA. Cancer screening: patient and population strategies. Med Clin North Am. 2023;107(6):989–99.
22. Park JM, Franken EA Jr, Garg M, Fajardo LL, Niklason LT. Breast tomosynthesis: present considerations and future applications. Radiographics. 2007;27(Suppl 1):S231–40.
23. Mukhtar TK, Yeates DR, Goldacre MJ. Breast cancer mortality trends in England and the assessment of the effectiveness of mammography screening: population-based study. J R Soc Med. 2013;106(6):234–42.
24. Marmot MG, Altman DG, Cameron DA, Dewar JA, Thompson SG, Wilcox M. The benefits and harms of breast cancer screening: an independent review. Br J Cancer. 2013;108(11):2205–40.
25. Costantini M, Belli P, Bufi E, Asunis AM, Ferra E, Bitti GT. Association between sonographic appearances of breast cancers and their histopathologic features and biomarkers. J Clin Ultrasound. 2016;44(1):26–33.
26. Shimizu H, Nakayama KI. A 23 gene-based molecular prognostic score precisely predicts overall survival of breast cancer patients. EBioMedicine. 2019;46:150–9.
27. Langley RR, Fidler IJ. The seed and soil hypothesis revisited – the role of tumor stroma interactions in metastasis to different organs. Int J Cancer. 2011;128(11):2527–35.
28. Da Costa D, Taddese A, Cure ML, Gerson D, Poppiti R Jr, Esserman LE. Common and unusual diseases of the nipple-areolar complex. Radiographics. 2007;27(Suppl 1):S65–77.

29. Babu B, Dev B, Mohanapriya T, Shalini CNS. Bilateral mammary Paget disease in a young adult female. Radiol Case Rep. 2018;13(3):586–91.
30. Sripathi S, Ayachit A, Kadavigere R, Kumar S, Eleti A, Sraj A. Spectrum of imaging findings in Paget's disease of the breast-a pictorial review. Insights Imaging. 2015;6(4):419–29.
31. Lam WW, Chu WC, Tse GM, Ma TK. Sonographic appearance of mucinous carcinoma of the breast. AJR Am J Roentgenol. 2004;182:1069–74.
32. Limaiem F, Ahmad F. Mucinous breast carcinoma. NCBI Bookshelf; 2023.

MIX
Papier aus verantwortungsvollen Quellen
Paper from responsible sources
FSC® C105338

If you have any concerns about our products,
you can contact us on
ProductSafety@springernature.com

In case Publisher is established outside the EU,
the EU authorized representative is:
Springer Nature Customer Service Center GmbH
Europaplatz 3, 69115 Heidelberg, Germany

Printed by Libri Plureos GmbH
in Hamburg, Germany